Stress and Breast Cancer

Stress and Breast Cancer

Edited by

Cary L. Cooper

Department of Management Sciences,
Institute of Science and Technology,
University of Manchester, UK

A Wiley Medical Publication

JOHN WILEY & SONS

Chichester · New York · Brisbane · Toronto · Singapore

Library of Congress Cataloging in Publication Data:

Stress and breast cancer.

   (A Wiley medical publication)
   Includes index
   1. Breast—Cancer—Psychosomatic aspects.
2. Stress (Psychology)   I. Cooper, Cary L.
II. Series.   [DNLM: 1. Breast Neoplasms—psychology.
2. Stress, Psychological.   WP 870 S915]
RC280.B8S78   1987   616.99′449071   87-19000
ISBN 0 471 91744 3

British Library Cataloguing in Publication Data

Stress and breast cancer.
   1. Breast—Cancer—Psychosomatic
   aspects.   2. Stress (Psychology)
   I. Cooper, Cary L.
   616.99′449   RC280.B8
   ISBN 0 471 91744 3

Phototypeset by Input Typesetting Ltd., London SW19 8DR.
Printed and bound in Great Britain.

Contributors

Cary L. Cooper
(*Editor*)
Department of Management Sciences, University of Manchester Institute of
Science and Technology, Manchester, UK.

Lea A. Baider
Department of Clinical Oncology and Radiotherapy, Sharett Institute of
Oncology, Hadassah University Hospital, Jerusalem, Israel.

Ursula C. Brandt
Department of Medicine, New England Deaconess Hospital, Harvard
Medical School, Boston, Massachusetts, USA.

David F. Cella
Department of Psychology and Social Sciences, Rush Presbyterian/St Luke's
Medical Center, Chicago, USA.

Alastair J. Cunningham
Division of Bio-research, Ontario Cancer Institute, Princess Margaret
Hospital, University of Toronto, Toronto, Canada.

Werner Georg
University of Giessen, West Germany.

Florian Hoffmann
University of Giessen, West Germany.

Robert S. Hoffman
Department of Psychiatry, UCLA and Medical Director of Psychosocial
Services, The Breast Center, Van Nuys, California, USA.

Jimmie C. Holland
Memorial Sloan-Kettering Cancer Center, New York, USA.

Da-Shih Hu
Department of Psychiatry, Dartmouth Medical School, Hanover, New Hampshire, USA.

Atara Kaplan-De-Nour
Department of Psychiatry, Hadassah University Hospital, Jerusalem, Israel.

Sandra M. Levy
Western Psychiatric Institute and Clinic, University of Pittsburgh, Pennsylvania, USA.

Jürgen Riehl
University of Giessen, West Germany.

Peter Schmidt
University of Giessen, West Germany

Peter M. Silberfarb
Department of Psychiatry, Dartmouth Medical School, Hanover, New Hampshire, USA.

Leo L. Stolbach
Department of Medicine, Division of Behavioral Medicine, Beth Israel Hospital, Harvard Medical School, Boston, Massachusetts, USA.

Basil A. Stoll
Department of Oncology, St Thomas' Hospital, London, UK.

Maggie Watson
CRC Psychological Medicine Group, The Royal Marsden Hospital, Surrey, UK.

Michael Wirsching
Clinic for Psychosomatic Medicine and Psychotherapy, School of Medicine, University of Giessen, West Germany.

Beverly D. Wise
Western Psychiatric Institute and Clinic, University of Pittsburgh, Pennsylvania, USA.

Contents

SECTION FOUR: BIOCHEMICAL PROCESSES AND
BREAST CANCER GROWTH

SECTION FIVE: INTERVENING AND COPING WITH
STRESS IN BREAST CANCER PATIENTS

SECTION SIX: METHODOLOGICAL CONSIDERATIONS IN
RESEARCH

Introduction

Throughout history, philosophers, physicians and scientists have suggested that there might be a link between life stress experiences and cancer. One of the earliest recorded is by Galen, who observed that cancer occurred more frequently in 'melancholic' than in 'sanguine' women. Further anecdotal evidence was furnished during the eighteenth and nineteenth centuries by such eminent physicians as Guy and Paget. The first scientific work became available with the publication by Herbert Snow (1893) of his book *Cancer and the Cancer Process*. He found that of the 250 successive patients examined at the London Cancer Hospital between 1883 and 1893 there had been 'immediate antecedent stress' in 156 (62.4 per cent). Thus, the first definite link connecting emotional stress with cancer was forged.

Since that time a large number of studies have been conducted on animal and human subjects (Cooper, 1984) exploring the relationship between psychosocial stress and cancer. In recent years, there has been a great deal of interest shown in the link between stress and breast cancer in particular, which probably mirrors the growing concern at the continuing increase in breast cancer. These studies reflect a wide spectrum of research interests, from an exploration of stress as a causal factor in the initiation and/or progression of cancer, to the physiological (i.e. the immune system) and psychological mechanisms moderating the link, to studies assessing the effectiveness of various counselling or other therapeutic techniques in minimizing the recurrence or progression of the disease. It is the purpose of this volume to bring together some of the leading researchers in the field to review the evidence available on the link between psychosocial stress and cancer, to help us understand the mechanisms in operation, to provide information about methods of treatment, and to discuss the methodological issues this research has raised.

The book is organized into several sections. The first section contains a brief overview chapter by Leo Stolbach and Ursula Brandt which highlights the main areas of research into psychosocial factors and breast cancer. They review four primary areas of research: psychosocial precursors of cancer, psychosocial factors and the progression of cancer, biological mediators of psychosocial effects, and interventions in breast cancer. This book will follow very closely this structure. The second section by Da-Shih Hu and Peter Silberfarb examines the extensive research evidence on the psychosocial stress *precursors* of breast cancer. The third section assesses the stress factors associated with the *progression* of breast cancer. In this section there are three chapters. Maggie Watson provides a brief overview of some of the major studies, with primary focus on England and Europe, while Sandra Levy and Beverly Wise explore some of the major US studies. There is also some overlap of studies between the two chapters in an effort to build conceptual models of the process of breast cancer development. The section is then rounded off by Michael Wirsching and his colleagues at the University of Giessen in West Germany in a long-term prospective study on the impact of psychosocial factors and breast cancer progression, which is a model of the kind of research approach that is needed in the future.

Section Four is comprised of a chapter by Basil Stoll on the biological mediators between the psychosocial stress factors and breast cancer growth. He explores the neuroendocrine and psychoendocrine influences on breast cancer development. Section Five examines the factors linked to treatment of and coping with breast cancer, and is composed of three chapters. The first by Alastair Cunningham assesses the research evidence on psychosocial interventions for breast cancer patients, exploring social support and coping strategies. The next chapter by Lea Baider and Atara Kaplan De-Nour examines the role of the family as a social support or moderating mechanism in the progression of breast cancer. This is a unique study in the field and provides fertile ground for further research. The final chapter in the section is by Robert Hoffman on the role of the psycho-oncologist in a breast cancer treatment centre. This highlights the possible role of psychologists and psychiatrists in the treatment of anxiety and psychological aspects of breast cancer, and how this might affect progression.

And finally, the last chapter by David Cella and Jimmie Holland explores the methodological issues one should consider, and take into account, in future research on the psychosocial stress factors related to the development and progression of breast cancer. It emphasizes some of the pitfalls of previous research and attempts to get us all on the 'right path' for future investigations in a growing and important field of endeavour.

REFERENCES

Cooper, C. (1984). *Psychosocial Stress and Cancer*, John Wiley & Sons, New York & Chichester.

Section One
Overview of Research

Stress and Breast Cancer
Edited by C. L. Cooper
© 1988 John Wiley & Sons Ltd

Chapter 1
Psychosocial Factors in the Development and Progression of Breast Cancer

Leo L. Stolbach[*†‡§]
and
Ursula C. Brandt[*¶**]

[*]*Division of Behavioral Medicine, The Charles F. Dana Research Foundation, The Thorndike Laboratory, Beth Israel Hospital, Boston, Massachusetts, and the Section on Behavioral Medicine, New England Deaconess Hospital, Boston, Massachusetts, USA*
[†]*Section of Hematology–Oncology, New England Deaconess Hospital, Boston, Massachusetts, USA*
[‡]*Department of Medicine, Harvard Medical School, Boston, Massachusetts, USA*
[§]*Department of Medicine, Boston University School of Medicine, Boston, Massachusetts, USA*
[**]*University of Witten/Herdecke, Medical School, Herdecke, West Germany*
[¶]*Department of Psychiatry, Harvard Medical School, USA*

1. BACKGROUND

The concept that the development or course of cancer may be affected by emotional factors has been repeatedly proposed throughout the recorded history of medicine. It is of considerable interest that many of the articles and books referring to this association have dealt with breast cancer, and in our review we will tend to focus on the reports and studies concerned with this disease. However, where appropriate, we will mention studies that deal with other cancers if they have served to establish psychosocial factors which may also be of relevance to breast cancer.

In the second century AD, Galen in *De Tumoribus* (Mettler and Mettler, 1947) stated that cancer was much more frequent in 'melancholic' than 'sanguine' women. During the eighteenth and nineteenth centuries, there were a variety of references to emotional factors related to cancer. These have been reviewed by Kowal (1955) and Mettler and Mettler (1947). Richard Guy (1759), in *An Essay on Scirrhous Tumors and Cancers*, described women prone to develop cancer as 'of a sedentary, melancholic disposition of mind, who meet with such disasters in life as occasion much trouble and grief'. The possibility that cancer could respond to hypnosis was reported by Sunderland in 1846 (see Gravitz, 1985) and Elliotson (1848). Nunn (1822), in a textbook *Cancer of the Breast*, emphasized that emotional factors influenced the growth of tumors of the breast and Walshe (1846), in his book *The Nature and Treatment of Cancer*, wrote: 'Much has been written on the influence of mental misery, sudden reverses of fortune and habitual gloominess of temper on the deposition of carcinomatous matter. If systematic writers can be credited, these constitute the most powerful cause of the disease; it would be vain to deny the facts of a very convincing character in respect to the agency of the mind in the production of this disease are frequently observed. I have myself met with cases in which the connection appeared so clear that I decided questioning its reality would have seemed a struggle against reason.'

James Paget (1870), in his textbook *Surgical Pathology*, stated that: 'The cases are so frequent in which deep anxiety, deferred hope and disappointment are quickly followed by the growth and increase of cancer, that we can hardly doubt that mental depression is a weighty addition to the other influences favoring the development of a cancerous constitution.' Subsequently, Snow (1893) reviewed the cases of 250 patients at the London Cancer Hospital. This report represented one of the first statistical analyses regarding the effects of psychological factors on the development of cancer. Snow stated that in 156 of the 250 patients studied, 'There had been immediately antecedent trouble, often in very poignant form as a loss of a near relative.' He concluded that 'The number of instances in which malignant disease of the breast and uterus follows immediately antecedent emotion of a depressing character is too large to be set down to chance, or to the general liability to the buffets of ill-fortune which the cancer patients, in their passage through life, share with most other people not so afflicted.'

During the first half of the twentieth century, there was a decrease in interest in the role of psychological factors in the development of cancer. However, Elida Evans (1926), a Jungian psychotherapist, reported on 100 cancer patients who underwent extensive psychotherapeutic evaluation after diagnosis. She described a common situation in cancer patients of an emotional relationship which had been broken off with no outlet for psychic energy.

LeShan and Worthington (1956), LeShan (1959) and Greer (1983) have provided excellent historical reviews regarding much of the early work on the role of emotional factors in the development and progression of cancer. These early studies are mainly anecdotal rather than scientific analyses of data obtained from clearly defined patient and control populations. However, the observations of possible psychological factors associated with cancer have been subsequently used to develop testable hypotheses which can be confirmed or rejected. In the early 1950s there emerged a renewed interest in the psychological characteristics of patients with cancer.

Blumberg, West and Ellis (1954), studying 50 patients at a Veterans Administration Hospital, reported that there was a significant difference in psychological characteristics, as determined by Minnesota Multiphasic Personality Interview (MMPI) scores, in patients with cancer who had rapidly progressive disease as compared to those with slower growing disease. Categorization of patients as showing fast or slow progression was determined separately for each type of cancer and was based on survival of plus or minus 50 per cent of the mean expected survival for the specific cancer. They described the rapidly progressing group as being 'consistently serious, over cooperative, over nice, over anxious, painfully sensitive, passive, apologetic personalities, who had suffered from this pitiful lack of self-expression and self-realization all their lives'. Even though this study was carried out in a Veterans Administration Hospital, it included four patients with breast cancer, but it is not stated whether they were men or women.

Bacon, Renneker and Cutler (1952) reported on the in-depth psychological evaluation of 40 patients with breast cancer and described the following patient characteristics: (1) masochistic character structure, (2) inhibited sexuality, (3) inhibited motherhood, (4) inability to discharge or deal with anger, aggressiveness or hostility covered over by a facade of pleasantness, (5) unresolved conflict with the mother handled through denial and unrealistic sacrifice and (6) delay in securing treatment. The patients included in this study were interviewed in a clinic setting at the Chicago Tumor Institute but the authors comment that the patients 'did not reflect the usual socioeconomic status of the clinic patients'. It is not possible to determine what criteria were used to select the patients for the in-depth psychological evaluation. In addition, it is not clear whether the characteristics described are generally applicable to breast cancer patients. The authors considered their work as exploratory and stated that further studies needed to be done to determine the role of 'emotional pressures as precipitating forces in the development of carcinoma', and that future work should be directed towards 'a deeper understanding of the role of normal and pathological emotional factors upon the body's defensive reaction to cancer'.

LeShan (1966) studied 450 cancer patients and 150 controls by the use of a projective test, the Worthington Personal History, and in some patients, intensive psychiatric interview. He reported that the cancer patients had a significantly higher incidence of a major loss early in life resulting in impaired ability to relate to others and finally another loss which resulted in feelings of hopelessness from six months to eight years prior to the diagnosis of cancer. It must be stated that the control population is not clearly defined.

These examples of early studies had a number of methodological flaws which included lack of controls or poorly defined control populations which were not truly comparable to the study populations (see Fox, 1978, 1982, 1983). Also, the effect of the knowledge of having a cancer on the responses of patients to the psychological tests was usually not taken into consideration. In addition, the appropriateness and interpretation of the psychological tests administered to these patients has been questioned. For instance, Fox (1983) examined twelve studies which involved prediction of survival or incidence of cancer, and which utilized the Minnesota Multiphasic Personality Interview (MMPI). In all of these studies, every one of the scales showed a relationship to cancer incidence, survival or relapse at least once and no scale showed such a relationship more than three times. Only one scale showed a consistent relationship in as many as three studies, namely a high score on the depression scale. Fox raises the question of whether the described associations could be due to chance rather than representing a truly significant association.

Both authors of the present chapter, in their respective oncologic and psychologic practices, have seen numerous patients who fit the described patterns of developing the initial manifestation of the cancer or its recurrence after a period of stress and/or significant loss. We also have seen patients with a strong positive attitude or a 'fighting spirit', who do much better than expected. Does this represent a selective recollection, on the part of the observer, of the extremes in any patient population or does an association of psychosocial factors with the development and progression of cancer indeed exist? The personal experience which we bring to the present inquiry needs to be placed into proper scientific perspective in order to develop testable hypotheses.

In our review, we will examine a number of prospective studies, prebiopsy studies and some retrospective investigations which may be relevant to either the development or the progression of cancer, with special emphasis on breast cancer. For more general overviews of the field we would refer the reader to a number of critical reviews (Fox, 1978, 1982, 1983; Cunningham, 1985; Greer, 1979, 1983; Bahnson, 1980, 1981; Perrin and Pierce, 1959; Crisp, 1970; Temoshok and Heller, 1984; Morrison and Paffenbarger, 1981).

2. PSYCHOSOCIAL PRECURSORS OF CANCER

There have been a number of studies which have examined large populations of individuals using a variety of psychological tests and interviews to evaluate premorbid psychological factors as they relate to cancer incidence. These factors will be separated into major categories and within each category we will examine studies which are prospective or retrospective separately.

Social Involvement

One of the best known prospective studies is that of Thomas, Duszynski and Shaffer (1979), who evaluated 1337 medical students at Johns Hopkins University from 1948 to 1964. These students were followed sequentially, and by 1979 20 of 913 white males whose data were analyzed for the report had developed a major cancer (excluding squamous and basal cell skin cancer, but not melanoma). A greater tendency for lack of closeness to parents, as measured by the Family Attitude Questionnaire, was found in the cancer group compared to the group who developed coronary heart disease and hypertension. In a follow-up report, Shaffer, Duszynski and Thomas (1982) reported an additional five cases of cancer, which brings the total number to 25 cases in the 913 subjects. The findings of the earlier report remained significant even when the samples were adjusted to account for cancer risk factors such as use of alcohol and/or tobacco and exposure to radiation. Unfortunately, we cannot use this information to define the premorbid characteristics of women who develop breast cancer since the percentage of women attending medical school during the study period was relatively small and the entire analysis in this study is limited to the men.

A recently reported study by Grassi and Milinari (1986), which included women with breast cancer, examined the role of parental relationships in 72 women presenting to the hospital with symptoms suggesting cancer. They studied 26 patients with breast masses and 46 with abnormal uterine bleeding. The patients completed the Family Attitude Questionnaire on the day of admission to the hospital prior to their surgery. Thirteen of the 26 women with breast masses were found to have cancer of the breast and 26 of the 46 with uterine bleeding were found to have uterine cancer. The combined cancer groups showed significantly less closeness to parents compared to the combined control group of 33 patients without cancer. The subset of patients with breast cancer showed a trend in the same direction for lack of closeness to parents but these results did not reach statistical significance. However, the breast cancer patients did show statistically significant negative attitudes towards the mother. The authors discuss a number of possible explanations for these results and conclude that 'some complex association involving many mechanisms exists between cancer and the affective and emotional climate in the family during early childhood. This area of research deserves more attention and requires further probing.'

The role of social isolation in the development of disease and mortality was examined by Berkman and Syme (1979) in a study of 6928 adults in Alameda County, California, who were initially evaluated in 1965. The age-adjusted relative risk for mortality for individuals who were most socially isolated was significantly higher than for those with the most social ties. This study did not report causes of death. However, a recent update of the data from the Alameda County cohort (Reynolds and Kaplan, 1987) evaluated the role of social contacts in the development of cancer. Measurements of social contact were based on a set of questions from the original 1965 questionnaire. The individuals were divided into quartiles on the basis of their responses and the quartile with least social contact was compared to that with the most social contact. Women who were socially isolated (reporting little contact with friends or relatives) were at significantly greater risk of dying of cancer of all sites. In addition, women who were both socially isolated and who reported that they felt isolated were at significantly greater risk of cancer incidence and mortality for all sites and for cancer mortality, but not cancer incidence for hormone-related sites including breast cancer.

Depression

The role of depression as a precursor to cancer has been examined by a number of investigators. One of the most widely quoted studies is that by Shekelle *et al.* (1981). This study correlates subsequent death from cancer over a seventeen-year period with higher depression scores on the MMPI test administered to 2020 male employees at a Western Electric plant at the initiation of the study. However, since it was limited to male employees, it cannot be used as evidence for the role of depression in breast cancer.

A larger study examining the role of depression in the development of cancer utilized the previously mentioned Alameda County database (Kaplan and Reynolds, 1987). The measure of depressive symptoms was based on eighteen items (see Roberts, 1981) selected from the original questionnaires administered in 1965. A total of 446 individuals developed 476 cancers (some individuals had multiple primaries) during the period 1966–1982. Seventy-six of 261 cancers in females were of the breast. There were 257 cancer deaths, and of the 134 female deaths 30 were due to breast cancer. Age-adjusted and multivariate analyses revealed an association between high levels of depressive symptoms at baseline and deaths from non-cancer causes with a *p* value of less than 0.001. However, there was no statistically significant association between either cancer incidence or cancer mortality and depressive symptoms for cancer of the breast or for all cancers. The authors of this study have compared their results to those reported by Shekelle for men at the Western Electric plant and have analyzed the differences between the two studies. They have been unable to develop a plausible explanation for the positive correlation with depression in Shekelle's study and the lack of an association reported in their study. They recommended further prospective studies to clarify this issue.

Greer and Morris (1975) examined the incidence of depression prior to the development of breast cancer and found that an equal percentage of cancer patients (35 per cent) and controls (36 per cent) with benign breast disease had been treated as outpatients for depressive illness in the five years preceding the first appearance of the breast lump.

In a well-balanced review of depression and cancer, Bieliauskas and Garron (1982) summarized the present information as follows: 'There is no solid evidence that cancer patients have increased depression in a psychiatric sense when compared to other patients, relatives, or normal control groups.' However, they also stated that 'Mild elevations in depressive symptomatology may be prospectively related to cancer incidence.' The latter statement was based mainly on the study of Shekelle *et al.* (1981) which, as mentioned before, was limited to males.

Stressful life events

A number of the early retrospective studies and numerous anecdotal reports suggested that stress or recent losses are associated with the development of cancer. LeShan and Worthington (1966) reported a psychological pattern of loss in early life followed by another significant loss in adult life as a precursor to the development of cancer. They did not give a breakdown as to the types of cancer which made up their cancer population. There also have been reports of significant losses in patients with lymphoma and leukemia (Greene, 1966) and lung cancer (Horne and Picard, 1979).

One of the few studies of breast cancer patients which correlated significant loss with the development of cancer is that of Becker (1986). He compared 71 breast cancer patients ('mostly Stage II') with 36 patients with fractures and 36 non-cancer patients, from a gynecological clinic, with regard to several psychosocial factors. All patients were under the age of 70. Questionnaires as well as a projective test and a clinical interview were used. He found more losses or upsetting events in childhood, and more frequent troublesome relationships, in his breast cancer patients than in the control groups. In addition, he studied life events in more detail by having his patients list the death of a close relative, psychosocial difficulties and illnesses in the first 20 years of their lives and in the past 20 years before diagnosis. He also classified their coping with these stressful events, according to his own categorization (Becker, 1982), into 'pathological' and non-pathological coping styles. He demonstrated poorer coping strategies in breast cancer patients than in the control groups. Compared to non-cancer patients, breast cancer patients differed less in the number of stressful events than in the way they reacted to these situations.

A number of the retrospective studies with positive results described above had major methodological flaws (see Fox, 1978, 1982, 1983; Greer, 1983). In contrast, a number of the more recent studies, carried out during the past 20 years, have generally not confirmed the hypothesis that stressful life events play a role in the development of breast cancer. A common format for these studies has been to test patients immediately prior to biopsy for a breast mass. At the time of the interview, neither the patient nor the interviewer knew with certainty whether the 'tumor' was benign or malignant.

Muslin (Muslin, Gyarfas and Pieper, 1966) was one of the first investigators to use this prebiopsy approach. A questionnaire was administered to all women admitted to the hospital for breast biopsy. The purpose of the questionnaire was to identify each woman's immediate relatives and close friends and to determine the time of permanent separations of the subject from any of these persons. Out of 165 admissions for breast biopsy, the investigators matched 37 patients with a malignant diagnosis and 37 with a benign biopsy. The results of this study did not reveal a higher frequency of recent or distant loss of emotionally important persons in the breast cancer patients compared with the matched benign controls.

Schonfield (1975) studied 112 Israeli women who were admitted for breast biopsy. Questionnaires, including the Holmes–Rahe Schedule of Recent Experience (Holmes and Rahe, 1967), were administered to these patients on the day prior to biopsy. Of the 112 women tested, 27 had malignant tumors and the remaining 85 had benign tumors. The results of this investigation revealed that the patients with the benign tumors had significantly greater life change scores. The authors state that this study does not support the premise that cancer patients have suffered greater significant losses during the years preceding the development of the malignant tumor. However, there has been considerable criticism of the life event instrument used in this study, including low reliability and validity as well as vagueness of many of the items (see Brown, 1981).

In a similar study, Greer and Morris (1975) interviewed 160 patients in the hospital on the day prior to biopsy. Using a structured interview, detailed information was obtained about the occurrence of stressful life events and the patients' characteristic modes of response to such events. The occurrence of previous stress was recorded in periods of five years and categorized according to the nature of the stressful event. At surgery, 69 of the patients were found to have breast cancer and 91 had a benign tumor. There was no statistically significant association between breast cancer and experience of stressful life events among the patients who had a diagnosis of cancer as compared to a benign tumor.

In a large case control study carried out through the Danish Cancer Registry, Ewertz (1986) examined the incidence of loss of a spouse and correlated it with the risk of developing breast cancer in 1792 cases of breast cancer and 1739 age-stratified randomly selected controls. There was no difference in the per cent of widows among the cancer patients as compared to the controls. Also, no difference was found between the two groups in the percentage of women who were divorced at the time of diagnosis.

Two other studies of stressful life events have compared patients with breast cancer to various control groups. The first of these by Snell and Graham (1971) compared 352 breast cancer patients and 670 controls. Comparisons were made concerning the extent to which the subjects and their immediate and extended families incurred such life events as death, divorce, illness, economic loss, residential mobility and feelings of being upset. Unfortunately, the control group was made up of a combination of patients with non-neoplastic diseases and patients with cancer of organs other than the breast or genitalia. The number of cancerous and non-cancerous diagnoses is not given in the description of the study. No difference was found between the breast cancer cases and the controls in the experiencing of either single events or cumulative numbers of events by the patients or members of their families. However, if one considers the possibility that the same life event factors which might be related to the development of breast cancer could also be associated with other cancers, then the use of patients with other cancers in the control group would minimize the potential differences between the two groups.

Priestman, Priestman and Bradshaw (1985) compared 100 breast cancer patients, 100 patients with benign diseases of the breast and 100 controls made up of friends and relatives of the patients as well as hospital personnel. Their study again failed to identify any relationship between an increase in life stress and the development of cancer.

The lack of correlation of stressful life events with the development of cancer reported in these studies may be somewhat surprising in view of the numerous anecdotal and retrospective reports in the literature suggesting such a correlation. One must keep in mind that there is considerable variability in the growth rates of different cancers. Therefore, the time periods selected for investigation of pertinent life events may not be relevant to the development of a particular cancer. Also, in many of these studies the reliability and validity of some of the instruments have been poor (see discussion by Brown, 1981). In addition, the importance of the life events to the patients has often been neglected. For this type of research, instruments which assess the significance of events for the individual have been proposed by Hurst, Jenkins and Rose (1978) and Cooper, Cooper and Faragher (1985).

Expression of emotions

Suppression of anger has emerged as a common theme in a number of studies of patients with breast cancer. For example, Greer and Morris (1975) and Morris *et al.* (1981) found significantly more suppression of anger in patients with breast cancer than in a control group of patients with benign breast disease.

Jansen and Muenz (1984) reported that patients with breast cancer tended to be less aggressive, less demonstrative, and had a decreased ability to express anger. However, the patients with cancer were considerably older and had a number of additional demographic dissimilarities when compared to those with fibrocystic disease and healthy women. These factors raise some doubts regarding the degree of confidence to be attached to this finding.

In contrast to these studies, Scherg, Cramer and Blohmke (1981) reported that a group of patients with breast cancer were comparable to healthy women without symptoms and to benign breast disease controls. These authors did not find a significant difference in suppression of anger and other factors, including anxiety.

Other Personality Characteristics

A prospective study which included females was carried out by Hagnell (1966). This study evaluated the personality characteristics of 2550 adults from a limited area in Sweden in 1947 and again ten years later. During this period 20 men and 22 women developed cancer. Of the 22 women with cancer nine had breast cancer. This represents too small a number to analyze separately. To summarize the findings of the study, Hagnell, using a scale developed by Sjöbring (1963), found a correlation between the personality characteristics of 'substability' and the risk of subsequent cancer in women but not in men. Substability is described as including such characteristics as warmth, heartiness, concreteness, industriousness, tendency to lose energy, and withdrawal from emotional expression when depressed. Fox (1978) has questioned whether these findings may have been the result of chance in view of the numerous subsets of characteristics analyzed. Also, Fox (1978) found, in reanalyzing the data, that 'mediostability' significantly protected women from later cancer, a result not reported by Hagnell.

Reynolds and Kaplan (1986) reported that 'unhappiness' is significantly associated with cancer incidence and mortality, based on the Alameda County cohort. In that cohort, 278 women developed cancer of whom 79 were diagnosed with breast cancer. Of the 144 women who died of cancer, 32 had breast cancer. Women who had described themselves as 'unhappy' were at greater risk for developing cancer, especially hormone-related cancers, than those more content with their lives. In addition, women who reported low life satisfaction showed greater mortality from hormone-related cancers.

Pauli and Schmid (1972) reported that patients with breast cancer had the following personality characteristics: hypochondriasis, depression, and exhibition of morbid anxieties, fears and phobias. The controls consisted of women who were postpartum and individuals who had a variety of benign diagnoses. The patients in the three groups were not well matched for age and this factor may have contributed to the reported psychological differences between the groups.

In a study of a number of psychological factors in patients who were admitted for a breast biopsy, Wirsching *et al*. (1982, 1985) found that patients with cancer tended to be inaccessible or overwhelmed when interviewed, showed emotional suppression, rationalization, little or no anxiety before the operation, demonstration of optimism, self-sufficiency, altruistic behavior and avoidance of conflicts. Predictions by the interviewer of diagnostic outcome, based on the psychological characteristics of the patients, were correct in 83 per cent of the eighteen cancer patients and in 71 per cent of the 38 patients with a benign diagnosis. An independent rater who did not interview the patients but only had the transcripts of the interview correctly predicted 94 per cent and 68 per cent of the diagnoses, respectively. Patients participating in this study were not asked about their own beliefs concerning the diagnosis.

An interesting study by Schwarz and Geyer (1984) addressed the question of patient knowledge of diagnosis prior to biopsy. Eighty-three women with tumors of the breast were interviewed prior to biopsy and were asked whether they thought the tumor was malignant or benign. The patients were able to predict the outcome of the biopsy with a fairly high degree of accuracy. Of the 23 patients who were found to have cancer, fifteen (65 per cent) made the correct diagnosis and of the patients whose tumor was found to be benign, 41 (77 per cent) correctly predicted the outcome. The respective rates of correct diagnosis by the patient's physician were 74 and 81 per cent.

Another interesting approach was taken by Engelman and Craddick (1984), who attempted to tap the 'unconscious symbolic relationships of patients to their cancer'. They used two projective tests, the Kahn Test of Symbol Arrangement and a Lifeline test. These were given to 146 tumor patients prior to breast biopsies. When compared to women with a benign biopsy, the women who were later diagnosed as having malignant tumors exhibited a knowledge of the diagnosis prior to biopsy based on the results of the projective tests. They also expressed the belief that the possibility of cure of the tumor was more remote. Both results were significant using multivariate analysis of variance that covaried with age. The findings were interpreted as showing an unconscious relationship between the mind and the body and were discussed in the context of the possible effects that negative beliefs might have on the disease and its treatment.

Prebiopsy studies have a design which clearly defines the timing of the interview. However, one has to consider the fact that many of the patients in these studies have received clues from their physician and from their own knowledge of their body (conscious and subconscious) and that this knowledge can affect the mood and attitudes measured by the investigator.

It is difficult from these studies to obtain a consistent pattern of a cancer-prone personality, especially in view of the fact that many of the studies were retrospective and the control populations were quite variable. Greer, Morris and Pettingale (1979) point out some of the problems in interpreting data obtained from patients with a known cancer diagnosis since the knowledge of the diagnosis can certainly affect the patient's mood and possibly the recollection of past events. Even in situations where the interview may be carried out prior to biopsy, there are often subtle or at times overt messages obtained by the patient from the physician which can indicate to the patient that the diagnosis of cancer is strongly suspected. In addition, there are probably both conscious and subconscious indicators of the likelihood of cancer being present which the patient incorporates and which again may affect the patient's mood and coping style.

3. PSYCHOSOCIAL FACTORS AND PROGRESSION OF CANCER

The question of whether the patient's attitude has an effect on prognosis has been studied by a number of investigators and has resulted in considerable controversy in the medical community.

Stress and Social Involvement

Funch and Marshall (1983) have examined the role of social stress and social involvement on survival. They studied 208 women with Stage I or Stage II breast cancer and 20 years later determined the length of survival of those women who had died. They analyzed the role of objective and subjective stress as well as the extent of social contact. Objective stress (death, illness or unemployment of a family member) was correlated with decreased survival for the oldest group of patients (66 years and older) and subjective stress (perceived tiredness or upset) was correlated with decreased survival for the youngest group (less than 45 years old). Concerning social support, women who had the least social contact had the shortest survival. This was true for the group less than 45 years old but not for the older age groups. As the authors point out, the instruments used to measure stress and social involvement were relatively crude and the study dealt only with the five-year period prior to the diagnosis of cancer. No information is available regarding these factors subsequent to that time. Also, the influence of these factors was relatively weak compared to such biological variables as stage of disease.

Attitudes Toward Cancer

The most compelling study, suggesting that attitude affects the outcome of patients with carcinoma of the breast, is that first reported by Greer, Morris and Pettingale (1979) and then updated by Pettingale *et al.* (1985). These investigators studied 57 women with Stage I and Stage II breast cancer three months after mastectomy. They administered a battery of psychological tests including a semistructured interview. On the basis of the interview, patients were divided into four categories: (1) denial, (2) fighting spirit, (3) stoic acceptance and (4) helplessness/hopelessness. The results, five years and ten years later, revealed a significantly better survival for patients with fighting spirit and denial compared to patients with stoic acceptance and helplessness/ hopelessness. Greer and Watson (1987) have recently validated a 40-item Mental Adjustment to Cancer questionnaire which can replace their more cumbersome semistructured interview and can be used to divide patients into the four attitude categories mentioned above. They have also added a new category of 'anxious preoccupation'. The use of this questionnaire should help other investigators to verify Greer's interesting findings.

In contrast to this study, a recent report by Cassileth *et al.* (1985) claims that psychosocial factors do not significantly affect outcome. The study reports the survival results for 204 patients with unresectable cancer of various sites and time to relapse for 55 patients with Stage I and II melanoma and 88 patients with Stage II breast cancer. The investigators utilized a self-report questionnaire which was composed of questions concerning seven variables which had been reported, in different studies, to be predictive of longevity or survival. These variables included social ties and marital history, job satisfaction, use of psychotropic drugs, general life evaluation/satisfaction, subjective view of adult health, degree of hopelessness/helplessness, and perception of the amount of adjustment required to cope with the new diagnosis. The authors report that in their study the social and psychological factors individually or in combination did not influence length of survival or time to relapse. One problem with this study is that selected questions from various psychological tests were summed into a psychosocial score. The only psychological instrument used in its entirety was the Beck Hopelessness Scale. The report also states that there was no correlation of psychosocial factors with major disease factors such as extent of disease and performance status. It is somewhat surprising that patients with limited disease (Stage I and II) would have similar psychosocial scores to patients with widely metastatic disease or that patients with performance status 0 (fully functional and without symptoms) would have equivalent scores to patients with performance status 4 (totally bedridden). If there is a lack of correlation between psychosocial scores and such disease factors, it is not unexpected that there would be no correlation with outcome. This study has been interpreted in an accompanying editorial and in articles in the lay press as showing that 'attitude' does not affect outcome. However, one has to question such an interpretation since many of the factors analyzed were measures of previous life experiences and satisfaction rather than attitude about life or the disease. We believe that it is premature to draw the authors' far-reaching conclusions from measures that we consider not to fulfill the minimal requirements of a standardized psychological test.

Mood and Emotional Distress

Weisman and Worden (1975) established 'survival quotients' for each of six cancer sites, including breast cancer, based on data from the Massachusetts Tumor Registry. This method allowed them to predict survival time for a particular cancer. The authors then compared 35 patients who had been psychologically evaluated, and subsequently died, with the 'normative' group (from the Tumor Registry) to determine which patients had survived shorter or longer periods than mean survival time. The patient's survival time was then correlated with psychological findings. Patients who lived significantly longer tended to maintain closer interpersonal relationships, to cooperate with the medical staff, to ask for and accept emotional support, and to experience less emotional distress than those with shorter survivals.

In contrast, Derogatis, Abeloff and Melisaratos (1979) found that in a group of 35 patients receiving chemotherapy for advanced breast cancer those patients who survived the longest showed considerably more psychological distress, in the form of anxiety, depression, guilt and hostility, as measured by the SCL90-R Symptom Checklist and the Affect Balance Scale. These same patients often were rated by their oncologists as being poorly adjusted and having poor attitudes. A major problem with this study is that the patients who fell into the short-term survivor category had received considerably more chemotherapy over a longer period of time and had a shorter disease-free interval since mastectomy. This would suggest that the short-term survivors had more advanced disease at the time of psychological testing. A number of subsequent reviews have interpreted the data of Derogatis as showing that the breast cancer patients who lived the longest were those who showed a 'fighting spirit'. This interpretation is not that given by Derogatis *et al.* (1979), who emphasize mainly the ability of the patients with longer survival to express negative emotions. These patient characteristics are quite different from the 'fighting spirit' described by Greer, Morris and Pettingale (1979) and Greer and Watson (1987), which is a much more positive and goal-oriented approach to dealing with one's disease.

In a recent study, Jamison, Burish and Wallston (1987) analyzed data from a group of 49 women with metastatic breast cancer who had previously been given a battery of psychological tests as part of several other studies. At the time of the analysis all 49 patients had died. They were divided into short-term and long-term survivors on the basis of a median split. No significant differences were found between the two groups on measures of mood (anxiety and depression), psychological adjustment, health value and self-esteem. The authors concluded 'that for breast cancer patients with metastatic disease, disease-related variables probably outweigh the influence of selected psychosocial factors in determining length of survival'. They do, however, suggest that the combined influence of certain interacting variables based on meaningful *a priori* predictions is more likely to generate findings between psychosocial factors and disease-related factors. This study is well designed and addresses many of the methodological flaws of earlier studies, but it deals with only a relatively small number of patients. It would have been useful to have had an analysis to determine the magnitude of difference required for a level of significance that would be clinically meaningful. It would also be interesting to determine if a comparison of the highest with the lowest quartile would show significant differences. A larger study of a similar population, taking into consideration the above concerns, would be useful.

Stoll (1976) studied 250 consecutive breast cancer patients and analysed their use of psychotropic drugs for anxiety or depression any time in the ten years prior to the diagnosis of cancer. This retrospective study showed that a significantly higher proportion of those who had required such treatment were found in two subsets of patients, namely those who had more advanced disease at the time of operation and those who showed evidence of recurrence within twelve months of initial surgery.

Levy (1984), in a study of a small group of breast cancer patients with metastases, found that patients whose disease was stable reported significantly more distress and unhappiness than the patients who subsequently died or those whose cancer was progressing. This study tends to confirm the observations of Derogatis *et al.* (1979).

Stavraky (1968) analyzed the course of 204 patients including 83 patients with breast cancer. Psychological tests were administered when the patient was first seen at the clinic. The clinical course was defined by dividing the survival of patients into quartiles. The patients with the most rapid course and the least rapid course were compared. The minimum of follow-up after testing was 40 months and the maximum 66 months. Stavraky's study did not confirm the finding that patients with a poor outcome showed the greatest degree of psychological abnormality. However, patients with the most favorable prognosis had the highest degree of underlying hostility or aggressiveness.

4. BIOLOGICAL MEDIATORS OF PSYCHOSOCIAL EFFECTS

The development, progression and regression of breast cancer is known to be influenced by hormonal factors. Selye (1950, 1980) originally described the effects of stress on the endocrine system and these findings have been confirmed in numerous animal and human studies. Therefore, hormonal factors represent logical mediators for the psychological effects on the course of breast cancer. The evidence regarding these hormonal effects is discussed in greater detail by Stoll in this book (see Chapter 6). Immunological factors have also been implicated in the development and progression of cancer, mainly from animal data but also from some human studies. The new field of 'psychoneuroimmunology' (see Solomon, 1985 and Locke *et al.*, 1985) attempts to present an integrated approach to mind–body interactions. There are also a number of interesting recent studies regarding possible mechanisms for 'communication' between the central nervous system and the immune system (see Blalock, Harbour-McMenamin and Smith, 1985; Besedovsky, del Rey and Sorkin, 1983; Ader and Cohen, 1985).

One example of the possible role of immune factors in breast cancer is the work of Levy *et al.* (1985). In a study of 75 patients with Stage I and Stage II breast cancer, they found that patients who had lower natural killer (NK) cell activity also had a higher incidence of positive nodes. In addition, patients who reported increased fatigue and lack of vigor and who complained of lack of family support tended to have significantly lower levels of NK cell activity. In contrast, patients who had higher NK cell activity appeared to be more distressed and maladjusted. One of the drawbacks of this study is that patients were interviewed prior to discharge from the hospital after either a mastectomy or segmental mastectomy. At that time the pathological information regarding the patient's nodes was probably known to the patient. This information, along with information regarding the additional treatment that might be necessary if the nodes were positive, could have affected the patient's basic attitude. Levy *et al.* (1987) have recently updated these results and have reported that NK cell values three months after initial evaluation were not affected significantly by intervening chemotherapy and/or radiation therapy. The association of distress factors with NK cell activity persisted at three months.

5. INTERVENTIONS IN BREAST CANCER

If one accepts the basic premise that psychological factors play a role in both the development and progression of breast cancer, then behavioral interventions would represent a logical approach. Cunningham (1985 and also in this book, see Chapter 7) has comprehensively reviewed the evidence for the role of psychological interventions. There is a major need for well-controlled prospective studies to determine the efficacy of behavioral interventions in improving not only the quality of life of patients with breast cancer and other malignancies, but also to increase the length of disease-free survival, overall survival and response to the standard forms of medical therapy.

The authors of the present chapter have carried out a feasibility study of behavioral interventions, including the relaxation response (Benson, Beary and Carol, 1974; Benson, 1984), for cancer patients. We are planning to further evaluate this approach in a prospective randomized study with special emphasis on breast cancer. We propose to study the short-term effects on mood and attitude and the possible long-term benefits as measured by improvement of outcome parameters such as survival.

CONCLUSIONS

In spite of numerous anecdotal reports and published studies regarding the role of psychosocial factors in the development of cancer, the present state of research in this area has not established a strong causal association between behavioral characteristics and human cancer. The studies to date have ident-ified possible psychological factors and life events which may contribute to the clinical development of cancer. In the case of breast cancer, these influ-ences may well be mediated through hormonal or immunological mechanisms but at present this is still conjectural. There is no evidence that psychosocial factors can initiate a tumor but, as discussed by Fox (1978), they may serve as promoters or accelerators of tumor growth.

The patient characteristics associated with cancer development in retro-spective studies are quite varied and data from different studies are often conflicting. Many of the studies have had serious methodological flaws and have not taken into consideration the significant lag period between the initiation of a cancer and its clinical detection. Also, in the retrospective studies, there is usually little information regarding the patient's mood and coping style in the years prior to the clinical appearance of the cancer. To quote Morrison and Paffenbarger (1981), most of the 'studies have failed to meet essential epidemiological criteria such as strong association, consistency, reproducibility, and specificity'.

The strongest supporting data for the role of psychosocial factors can be obtained from large prospective studies. Several of these have been described above. Lack of social support has been found to be a significant factor in several of the studies which included women who developed breast cancer. Hopefully, future data from these relatively large prospective studies will give them greater credibility and may also demonstrate other significant correlations which could confirm some of the associations made in retrospec-tive studies. The significant association of other factors such as depression and closeness to parents was observed in several prospective studies which were limited to men and these findings need further confirmation in women. Also, the findings of decreased ability to express emotions in breast cancer patients, which were based on prebiopsy studies, need to be confirmed in truly prospective studies.

Regarding the role of psychosocial factors in survival of patients with breast cancer, the following have been associated with longer survival:

1. 'Fighting spirit' or 'will to live'
2. Expression of emotions
3. Social contacts and support

However, as has been discussed earlier, the significance of these factors has not been consistently confirmed. There is a need for further studies in homogeneous patient populations. If the association of certain psychosocial variables with survival can be further substantiated, then interventions aimed at changing patient attitudes could play a role in improving prognosis.

GOALS FOR FUTURE RESEARCH

1. There is a need for well-designed prospective studies utilizing psychological instruments that have been well validated in cancer populations.

2. Studies should be carried out in clearly defined patient populations preferably of one disease site and careful attention should be given to factors such as stage of disease and age of patients. In studies of breast cancer patients, information regarding factors such as hormone receptor status should also be obtained.

3. Interventions aimed at changing attitudes which have been associated with a poor prognosis should be evaluated through prospective randomized studies, whenever possible.

4. Measurements of attitude, such as the Mental Adjustment to Cancer (Greer and Watson, 1987), which have been reported to be useful in determining prognosis, need to be validated in larger clearly defined patient populations.

Hopefully, this form of research will better delineate the patients who could be aided by changes in behavior and attitude. Such research should evaluate not only length of survival but also quality of life. In addition, a better understanding of the role of possible mediators in the development or progression of cancer can be very useful in possibly changing the course of the disease. Stoll (1979) aptly reviewed the role of hope as a factor in survival in a book *Mind and Cancer Prognosis* and we believe that the following passage is still applicable to our present state of knowledge:

We have no incontrovertible scientific evidence that emotional factors can influence the prognosis in the cancer patient—that is a question which still remains to be answered. However, to deny that such links exist is to deny numerous clinical observations in individual cases. Physicians are becoming increasingly conscious that the psychological state of the cancer patient deserves more attention than has been given to it in the past. Increasing interest in this field will not only improve the quality of life enjoyed by cancer patients, but it may also clarify the mechanism by which psychological factors appear to affect the duration of life in occasional cases.

ACKNOWLEDGEMENTS

We wish to thank Bernard Fox, PhD for his helpful advice and critique of this manuscript. We also wish to acknowledge Nile Albright, MD, Tenley Albright, MD and Hollis Albright, MD of the Advanced Medical Research Foundation and Herbert Benson, MD for their continuing advice and interest.

Preparation of this manuscript was supported in part by grant HL-22727 from the National Institutes of Health and grants from the Joan B. Kroc Foundation and the Ruth Mott Fund.

We also wish to thank Ms Youngsun Jung and Ms Ann Webster for invaluable help in preparation of the manuscript.

REFERENCES

Ader, R., and Cohen, N. (1985). CNS–immune system interactions: Conditioning phenomena, *Behav. Brain Sci.*, **8**, 379–394.

Bacon, C. L., Renneker, R., and Cutler, M. (1952). A psychosomatic survey of cancer of the breast, *Psychosom. Med.*, **14**, 453–460.

Bahnson, C. B. (1980). Stress and cancer: The state of the art. Part 1, *Psychosomatics*, **21**, 975–981.

Bahnson, C. B. (1981). Stress and cancer: The state of the art. Part 2, *Psychosomatics*, **22**, 207–220.

Becker, H. (1982). Das Mammakarzinom aus psychosomatischer, Sicht, Habil. Schrift, Heidelberg.

Becker, H. (1986). *Psychoonkologie*, Springer Verlag, Berlin.

Benson, H. (1984). *Beyond the Relaxation Response*, Times Books, New York.

Benson, H., Beary J. F., and Carol, M. P. (1974). The relaxation response, *Psychiatry*, **37**, 37–46.

Berkman, L. F., and Syme, S. L. (1979). Social networks, host resistance, and mortality: A nine year follow-up study of Alameda County residents, *Am. J. Epidem.*, **109**, 186–204.

Besedovsky, H. O., del Rey, A. E., and Sorkin, E. (1983). What do the immune system and the brain know about each other?, *Immunol. Today*, **4**, 342–346.

Bieliauskas, L. A., and Garron, D. C. (1982). Psychological depression and cancer, *Gen. Hosp. Psychiat.*, **4**, 187–195.

Blalock, J. E., Harbour-McMenamin, D., and Smith, E. M. (1985). Peptide hormones shared by the neuroendocrine and immunologic systems, *J. Immunol.*, **135**, 858s–861s.

Blumberg, E. M., West, P. M., and Ellis, F. W. (1954). A possible relationship between psychological factors and human cancer, *Psychosom. Med.*, **16**, 277–286.

Brown, G. W. (1981). Life events, psychiatric disorder and physical illness, *J. Psychosom. Res.*, 461–473.

Cassileth, B. R., Lusk, E. J., Miller, D. S., Brown, L. L., and Miller, C. (1985). Psychosocial correlates of survival in advanced malignant disease, *N. Engl. J. Med.*, **312**, 1551–1555.

Cooper, C. L., Cooper, R., and Faragher, B. (1985). Stress and life event methodology, *Stress Med.*, **1**, 287–289.

Crisp, A. H. (1970). Some psychosomatic aspects of neoplasia, *Brit. J. Med. Psychol.*, **43**, 313–331.

Cunningham, A. J. (1985). The influence of mind on cancer, *Can. Psychol.*, **26**, 13–29.

Derogatis, L. R., Abeloff, M. D., and Melisaratos, N. (1979). Psychological coping mechanisms and survival time in metastatic breast cancer, *J. Am. Med. Assoc.*, **242**, 1504–1508.

Elliotson, J. (1848). *Cure of a True Cancer of the Female Breast with Mesmerism*, Walton & Mitchell, London.

Engelman, S. R., and Craddick, R. (1984). The symbolic relationship of breast cancer patients to their cancer, cure, physician, and themselves, *Psychother. Psychosom.*, **41**, 68–76.

Evans, E. (1926). *A Psychological Study of Cancer*, Dodd-Mead, New York.

Ewertz, M. (1986). Bereavement and breast cancer, *Brit. J. Cancer*, **53**, 701–703.

Fox, B. H. (1978). Premorbid psychological factors as related to cancer incidence, *J. Behav. Med.*, **1**, 45–133.

Fox, B. H. (1982). A psychological measure as a predictor in cancer, in *Psychosocial Aspects of Cancer* (Eds J. Cohen, J. W. Cullen and L. R. Martin), Raven Press, New York.

Fox, B. H. (1983). Current theory of psychogenic effects on cancer incidence and prognosis, *J. Psychosoc. Oncol.*, **1**, 17–31.

Funch, D. P., and Marshall, J. (1983). The role of stress, social support and age in survival from breast cancer, *J. Psychosom. Res.*, **27**, 77–83.

Grassi, L., and Molinari, S. (1986). Family affective climate during the childhood of adult cancer patients, *J. Psychosoc. Oncol.*, **4**, 53–62.

Gravitz, M. A. (1985). An 1846 report of tumor remission associated with hypnosis, *Am. J. Hypnosis*, **28**, 16–19.

Greene, W. A. (1966). The psychosocial setting of the development of leukemia and lymphoma, *Ann. NY Acad. Sci.*, **125**, 794–801.

Greer, S. (1979). Psychological enquiry: A contribution to cancer research, *Psychol. Med.*, **9**, 81–89.

Greer, S. (1983). Cancer and the mind, *Brit. J. Psychiat.*, **143**, 535–543.

Greer, S., and Morris, T. (1975). Psychological attributes of women who develop breast cancer: A controlled study, *J. Psychosom. Res.*, **19**, 147–153.

Greer, S., Morris, T., and Pettingale, K. W. (1979). Psychological response to breast cancer: Effect on outcome, *Lancet*, **ii**, 785–7.

Greer, S., and Watson, M. (1987). Mental adjustment to cancer: Its management and prognostic significance, *Cancer Surveys*, in press.

Guy, R. (1759). *An Essay on Scirrhous Tumors and Cancers*, The Welcome Historical Medical Library, J. & A. Churchill, London.

Hagnell, O. (1966). The premorbid personality of persons who develop cancer in a total population investigated in 1947 and 1957, *Ann. NY Acad. Sci.*, **125**, 846–855.

Holmes, T. H., and Rahe, R. H. (1967). The Social Readjustment Rating Scale, *J. Psychosom. Res.*, **11**, 213–218.

Horne, R. L., and Picard, R. S. (1979). Psychosocial risk factors for lung cancer, *Psychosom. Med.*, **41**, 503–514.

Hurst, M. W., Jenkins, C. D., and Rose, R. M. (1978). The assessment of life change stress: A comparative and methodological inquiry, *Psychosom. Med.*, **40**, 126–141.

Jamison, R. N., Burish, T. G., and Wallston, K. A. (1987). Psychogenic factors in predicting survival of breast cancer patients, *J. Clin. Oncol.*, **5**, 768–772.

Jansen, M. A., and Muenz, L. R. (1984). A retrospective study of personality variables associated with fibrocystic disease and breast cancer, *J. Psychosom. Res.*, **28**, 35–42.

Kaplan, G. A., and Reynolds, P. (1987). Depression and cancer mortality and morbidity: Prospective evidence from the Alameda County study, *J. Behav. Med.*, in press.

Kowal, S. J. (1955). Emotions as a cause of cancer: Eighteenth and nineteenth century contributions, *Psychoanal. Rev.*, **42**, 217–227.

LeShan, L. (1959). Psychological states as factors in the development of malignant disease: A critical review, *J. Nat. Cancer Inst.*, **22**, 1–18.

LeShan, L. (1966). An emotional life-history pattern associated with neoplastic disease, *Ann. NY Acad. Sci.*, **125**, 780–793.

LeShan, L., and Worthington, R. E. (1956). Personality as a factor in the pathogenesis of cancer: A review of the literature, *Brit. J. Med. Psychol.*, **29**, 49–56.

Levy, S. M. (1984). Emotions and the progression of cancer: A review, *Advances*, **1**(1), 10–15.

Levy, S. M., Herberman, R., Lippman, M., and d'Angelo, T. (1987). Correlation of stress factors with sustained depression of natural killer cell activity and predicted prognosis in patients with breast cancer, *J. Clin. Oncol.*, **5**, 348–353.

Levy, S. M., Herberman, R., Maluish, A. M., Lippman, M., and Schlien, B. (1985). Prognostic risk assessment in primary breast cancer by behavioral and immunological parameters, *Health Psych.*, **4**, 99–113.

Locke, S. E., Ader, R., Besedovsky, H., Hall, N., Solomon, G. F., and Strom, T. (1985). *Foundations of Psychoneuroimmunology*, Aldine, Chicago.

Mettler, C. C., and Mettler, F. A. (1947). *History of Medicine*, Blakiston, Philadelphia.

Morris, T., Greer, S., Pettingale, K. W., and Watson, M. (1981). Patterns of expression of anger and their psychological correlates in women with breast cancer, *J. Psychosom. Res.*, **25**, 111–117.

Morrison, F. R., and Paffenbarger, R. A. (1981). Epidemiological aspects of biobehavior in the etiology of cancer, in *Perspectives on Behavioral Medicine* (Eds S. M. Weiss, J. A. Herd and B. H. Fox), Academic Press, New York.

Muslin, H. L., Gyarfas, K., and Pieper, W. J. (1966). Separation experience and cancer of the breast, *Ann. NY Acad. Sci.*, **125**, 802–806.

Nunn, T. H. (1822). *Cancer of the Breast*, J. & A. Churchill, London.

Paget, J. (1870). *Surgical Pathology*, 2nd edn, Longmans Green, London.

Pauli, H. K., and Schmid, V. (1972). Psychosomatische Aspekte bei der Klinischen Manifestation von Mamma-Karzinomen (Psychosomatic aspects in the clinical manifestation of breast cancers), *Z. Psychother. Med. Psychol.*, **22**, 76–80.

Perrin, G. M., and Pierce, I. R. (1959). Psychosomatic aspects of cancer, *Psychosom. Med.*, **21**, 397–421.

Pettingale, K. W., Morris, T., Greer, S., and Haybittle, J. L. (1985). Mental attitudes to cancer: An additional prognostic factor, *Lancet*, **i**, 750.

Priestman, T. J., Priestman, S. G., and Bradshaw, C. (1985). Stress and breast cancer, *Brit. J. Cancer*, **51**, 493–498.

Reynolds, P., and Kaplan, G. A. (1986). Psychological well-being and cancer, presented at the Annual Meeting of the Society for Epidemiologic Research, Pittsburgh, PA, June 1986.

Reynolds, P., and Kaplan, G. A. (1987). Social connections and risk for cancer: Prospective evidence from the Alameda County study, *Am. J. Epidem.*, in press.

Roberts, R. E. (1981). Prevalence of depressive symptoms among Mexican Americans, *J. Nerv. Ment. Dis.*, **169**, 213–219.

Scherg, H., Cramer, I., and Blohmke, M. (1981). Psychosocial factors and breast cancer: A critical reevaluation of established hypotheses, *Cancer Detection Prevention*, **4**, 165–71.

Schonfield, J. (1975). Psychological and life experience differences between Israeli women with benign and cancerous breast lesions, *J. Psychosom. Res.*, **19**, 229–234.

Schwarz, R., and Geyer, S. (1984). Social and psychological differences between cancer and non-cancer patients: Cause or consequence of the disease? *Psychother. Psychosom.*, **41**, 195–199.

Selye, H. (1950). *Stress*, Acta Inc. Med. Publishers, Montreal.

Selye, H. (1980). Correlating stress and cancer, *Am. J. Proct. Gastro. Col. Rect. Surg.*, **30**, 18–28.

Shaffer, J. H., Duszynski, K. R., and Thomas, C. B. (1982). Family attitudes in youth as a possible precursor of cancer among physicians: A search for explanatory mechanisms, *J. Behav. Med.*, **5**, 143–163.

Shekelle, R. B., Raynor, W. J., Ostfeld, A. M., Garron, D. C., Bieliauskas, L. A., Liu, S. C., Maliza, C., and Oglesby, P. (1981). Psychological depression and 17 year risk of death from cancer, *J. Psychosom. Med.*, **43**, 117–125.

Sjöbring, H. (1963). *La Personalité, Structure et Dévelopment*, Doin, Paris.

Snell, L., and Graham, S. (1971). Social trauma as related to cancer of the breast, *Brit. J. Cancer*, **25**, 721–734.

Snow, H. L. (1893). *Cancer and the Cancer Process*, J. & A. Churchill, London.

Solomon, G. F. (1985). The emerging field of psychoneuroendocrinology, *Advances*, **2**(10), 6–19.

Stavraky, K. M. (1968). Psychological factors in the outcome of human cancer, *J. Psychosom. Res.*, **12**, 251–259.

Stoll, B. A. (1976). Psychosomatic factors and tumor growth, in *Risk Factors in Breast Cancer* (Ed B. A. Stoll), Heinemann Medical, London.

Stoll, B. A. (1979). Is hope a factor in survival? in *Mind and Cancer Prognosis* (Ed. B. A. Stoll), John Wiley, London, pp. 183–197.

Temoshok, L., and Heller, B. (1984). On comparing apples, oranges, and fruit salad: A methodological overview of medical outcome studies in psychosocial oncology, in *Psychosocial Stress and Cancer* (Ed. C. L. Cooper), John Wiley, London.

Thomas, C. B., Duszynski, K. R., and Shaffer, J. W. (1979). Family attitudes reported in youth as potential predictors of cancer, *Psychosom. Med.*, **41**, 287–302.

Walshe, W. H. (1846). *The Nature and Treatment of Cancer*, Taylor & Walton, London, p. 155.

Weisman, A. D., and Worden, J. W. (1975). Psychosocial analysis of cancer deaths, *Omega*, **6**, 61–75.

Wirsching, M., Hoffmann, F., Stierlin, H., Weber, G., and Wirsching, B. (1985). Prebioptic psychological characteristics of breast cancer patients, *Psychother. Psychosom.*, **43**, 69–76.

Wirsching, M., Stierlin, H., Hoffmann, F., Weber, G., and Wirsching, B. (1982). Psychological identification of breast cancer patients before biopsy, *J. Psychosom. Res.*, **26**, 1–10.

Section Two
Psychosocial Precursors to Breast Cancer

Stress and Breast Cancer
Edited by C. L. Cooper
© 1988 John Wiley & Sons Ltd

Chapter 2
Psychological Factors: Do They Influence Breast Cancer?

Da-Shih Hu
Assistant Professor of Psychiatry, Director, Psychiatric Emergency Service
and
Peter M. Silberfarb
Professor of Psychiatry and of Medicine, Chairman, Department of Psychiatry, The Dartmouth Medical School and the Norris Cotton Cancer Center, Dartmouth–Hitchcock Medical Center, Hanover, New Hampshire, USA

'I didn't know enough then to believe that stress could make you ill.' (Jill Ireland, actress, speaking of her breast cancer in *Parade Magazine* (Seligson, 1987))

There is no question that the idea that psychological variables can influence the development and prognosis of cancer appeals to the public. Articles appear in the popular press. Books like Simonton's *Getting Well Again* (Simonton, Matthews-Simonton and Creighton, 1978) and LeShan's *You Can Fight For Your Life* (1977) attract attention from the media and find their way into the discussions of cancer support groups because of the hope they offer with their advocacy of the psychological changes cancer patients can make to improve their prognoses. To some degree this is undoubtedly a manifestation of the human need to make order out of randomness. As Harold Kushner writes in *When Bad Things Happen To Good People*, 'We could bear nearly any pain or disappointment if we thought there was a reason behind it, a purpose to it. But even a lesser burden becomes too much for us if we feel it makes no sense' (1981, p. 135). Nevertheless, the overwhelming public interest in the possibility of combatting cancer by psychological strategies dictates that anyone with interest in the cancer field have an awareness of how much legitimacy there is to these tantalizing offers of prolonged life.

A review of the literature reveals striking contrasts in the scientific reception accorded this idea. Standard oncology texts rarely address the question

27

of psychological stress and cancer or the cancer-prone personality; researchers in the field have even reported experiencing negative or resistant attitudes towards such inquiry (Booth, 1965). On the other hand, some of what has been written in support of the idea exudes such fervor that one feels it is uneasily close to proselytizing. That there should be so few middle-ground opinions emphasizes the importance of the physician's remaining receptive to exploring both sides of the question.

This chapter will attempt to undertake such a balanced inquiry, particularly with regard to how psychological matters may influence the development and growth of breast cancer. Much of the literature, however, does not distinguish breast cancer from other cancer in this regard, so that some of the discussion will inevitably also focus on psychological connections with cancer in general.

THE EARLY OBSERVATIONS

Several writers (Kowal, 1955; LeShan and Worthington, 1956) have reviewed earlier medical writings on the subject, and the reader is directed to them for a fuller discussion. Suffice it to say that there have been those in the medical field who have postulated a connection between psychological factors and cancer going back several centuries, and that the predisposing factors noted most often seemed to be related to emotions, particularly grief and despair.

As a brief aside, it should be noted that many authors, reviewing the literature, state that even Galen writing in the second century AD, pointed to the connection between cancer and melancholic humor. However, it is not always clear that his cancer and our cancer are the same thing (Rather, 1978, p. 9); moreover, melancholic humor referred to the fluid black bile and not to a temperamental style. While Galen does attribute both cancer and melancholy to an excess of black bile, he does not appear to have stated that the two were any more directly connected than to have a common underlying cause. (Among the other things he attributed to an excess of *melan chole*, black bile, were fever, schistosomiasis, anthrax, ileus and leprosy (Siegel, 1968).)

In his extensive survey, *The Genesis of Cancer*, Rather (1978) notes that the earliest reference to a direct connection between emotions and cancer is from Johannes Pechlin, a seventeenth-century physician who embraced the prevailing humoral theory of the day. He felt there was a connection between fear and sorrow and the malignant transformation of breast tumors. From this time, though the theories of oncogenesis changed, the possible associ-ation with emotions remained. Gendron, who broke with humoral tradition to suggest a solidistic lymphatic theory of oncogenesis in the early 1700s, noted the influence of fright and grief (Kowal, 1955). When humoral theory had been modified to the lymphatic humoralism that was to dominate eight-eenth-century thought, Boerhaave noted sad and bilious emotions as a contributory cause of cancer.

This viewpoint was so well developed that Walshe, writing within a decade of the introduction of the cell theory of cancer, was already stating in his classic book *The Nature And Treatment Of Cancer* (1846) that among the acquired predisposing causes to cancer were both temperament (women of 'high colour and sanguineous temperament' were 'more subject to mammary cancer') and mental affliction, though of the latter he adds 'the extent to which this influence works practically, (*sic*) has doubtless been overestimated (pp. 153–5)'.

Since the nineteenth century the literature has been scattered with references to such phenomena, though modern authors have tended to overlook the fact that the relationship was not always seen as a direct causal one. Paget, for example, noted by different writers including both LeShan and Kowal to have mentioned the link, does indeed say in his *Lectures On Surgical Pathology* (1871), 'we can hardly doubt that mental depression is a weighty addition to the other influences that favour the development of the cancerous constitution', but he goes on to add, 'I do not at all suppose that it could of itself generate a cancerous condition of the blood . . . it is consistent with the many other facts showing the affinity between cancer and depressed nutrition (p. 800).' Certainly the development of cancer is a multifactorial phenomenon, and any theory of psychological causality needs to recognize this. As the above example demonstrates, there is a tendency to overinterpret the literature and to underrepresent the complexity of the issue.

It would be well, then, before starting a review of the studies regarding the connection between psychological factors and breast cancer, to develop an understanding of the natural history of breast cancer, as this has a bearing on understanding the possible relationships between the two. Only certain relevant areas will be explored here; the reader is referred to a general source for a fuller discussion (e.g. Harris *et al.*, 1985).

THE (SELECTED) NATURAL HISTORY OF BREAST CANCER

There are a number of risk factors for breast cancer that may reflect some influence of psychological factors. One of the most striking and consistently noted is that there is a wide range of incidence rates and mortality rates across geographic regions, the rates in low-risk areas, notably Asia, being up to six or more times lower than in high-risk areas, notably the United States and Europe. That this is not due to genetic factors but to environmental ones is generally accepted and supported by several lines of evidence: the incidence rates of women of Asian descent rise over several generations after immigration to the United States and approach those of Caucasian women, and the mortality from breast cancer has risen dramatically in Japan since World War II and the encroachment of western culture (Moore, Moore and Moore, 1983; Ketcham and Sindelar, 1975).

Just what environmental factors these are has not yet been determined. Nevertheless the difference has been so striking that Stefansson devoted a book, *Cancer: Disease Of Civilization* (1960) to his and others' observations that cancer of all types is rare among more primitive people and that its appearance seems to be associated with the influx of civilization (at least western civilization). He cites diet as a possible major cause of this. Of course other theories could be advanced, for example, this observation would also be consistent with psychological stress being a component in the etiology of cancer.

There are many other risk factors noted for breast cancer (Ketcham and Sindelar, 1975; Miller and Bulbrook, 1980; Moore, Moore and Moore, 1983). A number could be seen as related to psychological factors, though there are obviously many other possible explanations. These include (1) marital status, single women having a greater risk than married (perhaps regardless of parity), (2) socioeconomic class, women in higher SEC having a greater risk, (3) education, women with higher education having a greater risk and (4) hormonal influences.

There is general acknowledgement that the development of breast cancer is related to hormonal environment, but which hormones are how important for this has yet to be determined. Higher estrogen levels, higher prolactin levels, lower progesterone levels and lower androgen levels have all been suggested to play a role in the expression of breast cancer, but the extent of their effects is still conjectural—for example, although postmenopausal exogenous estrogens increase breast cancer risk, there has not been any such increase found in women taking oral contraceptives (Harris *et al.*, 1985). Nevertheless, there is clearly the possibility that psychoendocrine factors could be a possible link between stress and breast cancer.

Another risk factor that is still a matter of controversy is benign breast disease. Studies have indicated for some time that there is a two- to threefold increased risk in women so affected. More recent examinations of the data suggest that perhaps only epithelial hyperplasia is a risk factor; again this awaits further clarification. The implication of this for research on breast cancer risk is that women with benign breast disease may not be suitable as controls for breast cancer patients (since whatever operates to increase the risk of breast cancer may do so by a mechanism that stimulates benign disease), something which is done in several studies.

Some of the difficulty about adequately defining these risk factors, let alone the role of psychological factors, may stem from the fact that breast cancer is not a unitary disease. There are at least eight histologic pure tumor groups of breast cancer, as well as combinations of these (Harris *et al.*, 1985). Henderson and Canellos (1980a) suggest that, even within Stage I carcinoma, there are three subgroups with varying degrees of aggressiveness and metastatic potential. Studies about the psychological interplay with breast cancer rely on the assumption that there is some factor which may be operative in enough of these varied types of breast cancer to show up in a sampling of breast cancer patients, or that whatever is felt to be the important factor operates regardless of the disease's diversity. Unfortunately, as Henderson and Canellos (1980b) point out, 'the overinterpretation of small, uncontrolled, and poorly designed studies or the extrapolation from the experience of an individual practitioner will usually be misleading'. This is applicable not only for the medical researchers to whom it was aimed, but also for psychological researchers.

Regarding the development of a breast tumor, there are several salient points for the psychological investigator. For one, it has become increasingly evident that there are multiple stages to the development of a cancer. The simplest schema proposes a two-step process: initiation, where cells are irreversibly changed into potentially neoplastic cells by an alteration in the genetic material of the cell, and promotion, where agents act that facilitate the altered genetic information's being expressed, i.e. promote growth of the already initiated cell line (Pitot, 1985). Although this was developed with regard to chemical carcinogenesis, it can be used as a skeleton for carcinogenesis in general, keeping in mind that other kinds of carcinogenesis may be even more complex. Is the hypothesized role of stress in the development of breast cancer one of initiator or of promoter? It is hard to imagine a pathway by which stress could actually alter cellular DNA. There are, however, many ways in which abnormal cell growth could be facilitated. Therefore, it is much more sensible to view stress as a potential promoter. Sklar and Anisman (1981), following a similar line of reasoning, reach a similar conclusion.

Psychological factors acting as promoters could potentially exert very powerful effects on the genesis and growth of clinical cancer. With breast cancer in particular there is strong evidence that promotion plays a major role in the expression of the neoplasm. In general, there seems to be a much higher incidence of neoplastic mammary cells than is ever manifested clinically. In women who develop breast cancer, it is well known that there is a high incidence of multicentricity (Harris *et al.*, 1985). In one study, 13.4 per cent of women with breast cancer had one or more other independent cancers elsewhere in the same breast. About 15 per cent of women with cancer will also be found to have cancer in the contralateral breast on biopsy. Yet the prevalences of synchronous unilateral, synchronous bilateral or metachronous bilateral tumors are much less than any of these figures would suggest they ought to be. Even more impressively, autopsy studies indicate that 25–30 per cent of *all* women have either *in situ* or invasive breast malignancies, far in excess of the number ever actually manifested (Andersen, Nielsen and Jensen, 1985). All of these lines of evidence suggest that many more neoplastic cells actually develop than ever present as clinical disease.

Even with metastases, the presence of neoplastic cells does not necessitate the appearance of clinical disease. Breast tumors have the potential to metastasize by the time they are 0.06 cm in diameter, and if a tumor is going to metastasize, in general it will already have done so by the time the tumor is clinically detectable (Fournier *et al.*, 1985). One study found through special histologic techniques that 24 per cent of women who would have been regarded as having Stage I disease actually had micrometastases (less than 2 mm in diameter) in axillary lymph nodes. These women had no significant difference in survival rate from those who had no detectable evidence of metastatic involvement, implying that the course of their disease was determined not just by whether their disease had spread but also by how well the spread flourished. Obviously then, there are body conditions that are more and less conducive to the growth of breast cancer, and it would be reasonable to suppose that psychological factors could have an effect on these.

One final aspect of the natural history of breast cancer concerns doubling time, the amount of time needed for a tumor mass to double in size. Various calculations have been made of this for breast cancer, and show a wide range from days to one and a half years, with an average of about four months (Devitt, 1976). If a tumor cell were to grow constantly at the last rate, it would take about eight years to become clinically evident, and some sources suggest an even longer doubling time with a time span of 15–20 years to become clinically evident (Fournier *et al.*, 1985). The obvious bearing that this has on psychological research related to breast cancer is that any hypothesis suggesting specific incidents or emotions causing the disease would have to consider events and traits from at least a decade before the diagnosis was made. And any event that exerted an effect for only a short period would not appreciably decrease the time it took for a cancer to become evident and therefore would not increase the risk of cancer.

The evidence cited above suggests that by the time a breast cancer is found, even if at a clinically early stage, it is already biologically late in its development (Fournier *et al.*, 1985). Any psychological factor that would be supposed to affect the cancer after it is found would potentially have had the chance to affect the same disease in the same way for years before its discovery and even have a role in its becoming discoverable.

The natural history of breast cancer suggests the following about psychological factors. (1) They probably operate (if they operate) as promoters of cancer rather than as initiators. That being so, if they do affect the manifestation of breast cancer, they probably affect the progression of breast cancer in the same way, i.e. *the questions of whether psychological factors can influence the development of cancer and whether they can affect the prognosis of breast cancer are the same question.* It appears that this notable point has frequently been overlooked in the published literature. (2) Because it is likely that promotion is clinically important in the manifestation of breast cancer, stress as a promoter could in fact be clinically important in the manifestation of breast cancer. (3) Nevertheless, the variability of the disease means that psychological factors that affect only a subpopulation of breast cancer patients may be demonstrable only inconsistently in studies done on an unselected population. (4) Any such factors would have to be operative a goodly number of years before the cancer appeared, and for a sizable period of time.

THE POSTULATED PSYCHOLOGICAL VARIABLES

With the above in mind, a consideration can now be given to some of the studies that have been undertaken to specifically explore the relationship between psychological stresses and breast cancer. It seems best to present them in chronological order. From that will be seen the progression in study methods, from general retrospective impressions to statistical analyses to controlled prospective studies. Yet with all of them there are design flaws, due more perhaps to the difficulty of mounting an unassailable research project on such a complex topic than to laxity on the authors' part.

This problem of methodology has been addressed in a number of papers (Perrin and Pierce, 1959; LeShan, 1960; Fox, 1976; Greer and Morris, 1978). Among the difficulties noted are: (1) the problems with defining appropriate study and control groups, (2) the selection of measurement tools that are valid and reliable but still useful, (3) the need for thoughtful application of statistical tests, (4) the importance of using well-defined or universally understood terminology, and (5) the impossibility of demonstrating that findings in retrospective studies did not occur as a consequence rather than an antecedent of the disease. Even prospective studies, such as evaluating women who are having a breast biopsy, may be influenced by women having some idea of whether their breast mass is malignant through unconscious cues picked up from their physician or their own bodies. Fox further makes a distinction between true prospective studies and anterospective studies, where subjects are still chosen on the basis of their having developed cancer even though the data analyzed are from before they were known to have cancer. The majority of 'prospective' cancer studies fall into the latter category. Of course, one further difficulty is the controlling of or even adjusting for all the variables that are known to biologically affect the process of cancer: especially with the many other factors affecting the disease, the effect of psychological factors may be real but not always demonstrable. That no study is inarguable must be a given in such a complex area.

Although this chapter is targeted at breast cancer, there are a number of papers that attempt to describe a personality or life history common to cancer patients of all types, and, since this obviously includes such a common cancer as breast carcinoma, these will also be reviewed. Finally, as noted at the end of the above section, a full consideration suggests that the question of interaction of psychological variables with prognosis is not a separate one, and studies bearing on that will be considered too.

The two major schools of thought about what psychologically might influence the growth of cancer suggest either (1) that there are certain personality traits which predispose someone to cancer or (2) that there is a certain group of life events that does the same thing. Some authors suggest that both are true.

THE STUDIES

The earliest studies to explore the connection of psychological factors to cancer were compilations of personal observation. In 1926 Evans (cited in LeShan, 1959), based on her Jungian psychotherapy with 100 cancer patients, concluded that the cancer patient typically had lost an important emotional relationship prior to developing the cancer, though over what time period is unclear. She suggested that this loss led to the patient's turning his psychic energy inward, where it was expressed as a cancer. Another report based on similarly obtained data was Wilhelm Reich's 1948 discussion of the cancer biopathy (cited in Dew, 1981). He felt that cancer patients had a preexisting emotional and characterologic resignation and that this manifested itself in a chronic emotional calm. To him, this was an outward manifestation of a biological energy depletion.

In 1951, Tarlau and Smalheiser published the first paper that used 'objective' psychological data to examine the connection between cancer and psychological variables. They interviewed, administered Rorschachs to and obtained human figure drawings from 22 women, eleven with breast cancer and eleven with cervical cancer. From these they concluded that the patients generally had come from mother-dominated families and had rejected their femininity in consequence. The breast cancer patients, in particular, adapted by denying their sexuality. They were felt to be functioning at a primitive oral level, where they severely repressed their emotional life but manifested little overt anxiety. As there was apparently no control group, this analysis, though supported by data, was really of an impressionistic nature.

In 1952, Cobb, in a doctoral dissertation (cited in LeShan and Worthington, 1956), interviewed and administered projective tests to 100 patients with different types of cancer. She concluded that, in general, they reported more negative reactions to their families, tended to withdraw under stress, and seemed to regard emotional involvement as dangerous and avoided it. Cobb compared some of these data with control groups made up of the general population and of colitis patients.

The same year, Bacon, Renneker and Cutler studied 40 breast cancer patients using a dynamic evaluation based on Alexander's work and concluded that they showed a masochistic character structure, inhibited sexuality, inhibited motherhood, an unresolved hostility towards their own mothers and an inhibited ability to express anger. The thing they found most commonly in recent precancerous history was a feeling of increasing guilt over the year preceding the discovery of the cancer. Yet they hasten to point out that 'we would like to avoid the formation of a picture of "the woman with cancer of the breast" . . . inroads into this (problem) . . . will only continue so long as we keep our focus on the individual . . . It should also be emphasized that we are not attempting to present the hypothesis that only emotional factors form the long chain reaction which leads to cancer' (p. 454). Such a balanced view could serve well for all investigators in the field.

The next major paper was Blumberg, West and Ellis' (1954), where, based on their observation of the 'polite apologetic, almost painful acquiescence of the patients with rapidly progressing disease . . . contrasted with the more expressive and sometimes bizarre personalities of those who responded brilliantly to therapy' (p. 277), they administered a battery of psychological tests to 50 cancer patients with contrasting courses. However, they decided to use only MMPI data for analysis, and described a pattern which correctly identified patients as good or poor treatment responders 78 per cent of the time. They made no attempt to subsequently verify these patterns on a group of patients who were not originally in the study, confounding any test for statistical significance. The patients with rapid progression of disease had scores suggesting a tendency to cover inner distress with outward calm and an inability to relieve anxiety or depression through normal patterns of discharge.

An attempt to crossvalidate the Blumberg *et al.* study was done by Krasnoff (1959). He, however, restricted his study to one type of cancer (malignant melanoma) and used specific normative survival data to define fast and slow progression of disease. The patients were given Rorschachs and MMPIs. Neither test served to differentiate the two groups. The fast group was, however, significantly lower in socioeconomic class and verbal intelligence than the slow group.

Reznikoff (1955) gave TATs, sentence completion tests and a series of family-related questionnaires to 50 women who had come to a clinic for evaluation of a breast mass and 25 normal women. Half of the women with breast masses subsequently proved to have malignancies. Whether these groups were otherwise equivalent demographically is not stated; in fact, one variable that is mentioned is that the normals were in general from a higher socioeconomic class, clearly contrary to normal expectations. The author's conclusions were that the breast cancer women, as compared to the normals, reported a greater number of sibling deaths at an early age, had had childhoods entailing more responsibility, especially caring for younger children, and expressed more negative attitudes about pregnancy, birth and their feminine identification. Benign patients differed much less markedly. One wonders how much the results reflect an unspoken feeling of psychosomatic specificity by the investigator, that the location of the cancer was reflective of the patients' psychological conflicts, a general idea that is found particularly in these earlier studies.

In what was essentially an extended case report into the uses of hypnosis with cancer, Butler (1954) described cancer patients as those who fail to express themselves and suffer with self-pity and stoicism. He adds, rather cryptically, that one of the advantages of hypnosis is that 'life is prolonged', but gives little evidence for that in the body of the work. Nevertheless, if this is indeed what he meant to say, he is one of the earliest writers to espouse what has become a more prevalent view, at least among cancer patients, that there are things that they can do psychologically to improve their prognoses.

Sixty women, 20 each with breast cancer, cervical cancer and no cancer, were given a series of psychological tests by Wheeler and Caldwell (1955) in an attempt to replicate the Tarlau and Smalheiser study with the addition of controls. For the most part, they found no striking differences among the groups, either corresponding to the Tarlau and Smalheiser or Bacon, Renneker and Cutler studies, although there was a statistically significant but small trend for cancer patients to have more sexual conflicts. Women with cervical cancer did seem to have more disturbed family backgrounds than the others (the authors noted that this could be mediated by those patients being more sexually active because they sought more affection from others), but those with breast cancer had, if anything, closer mother–daughter ties than either of the two other groups.

LeShan and Worthington entered the field in 1955 with a report on 152 patients with cancer and 125 controls who had been given a projective questionnaire called the Worthington Personal History. These were evaluated, largely subjectively it appears, and found to show a pattern among cancer patients of the loss of an important relationship before the diagnosis of the cancer (no actual time frame was given, though one example is three years before), an inability to express hostile feelings, and tension over the death of a parent, usually far in the past. An attempt by the authors to predict who had cancer among 28 records obtained later led to correct predictions in 24 of them. This study was followed in 1956 by a report on 250 patients using the same instrument. An additional feature of cancer patients, a marked amount of self-dislike, was noted, and it was remarked that the loss of a major relationship occurred from six months to eight years before the appearance of the tumor. Given what has already been said about the length of time needed for a tumor to become apparent, one might wonder about the effect of having cancer on retrospective recall of major losses as reasonably as one might wonder about the effect of a recent major loss on the development of cancer.

In an unusual follow-up to this paper, the authors (LeShan and Worthington, 1956) made a series of predictions concerning previously collected data. These were (1) that cancer mortality rates by marital status should be widowed>divorced>married>single, (2) that married individuals with children should have lower cancer mortality rates than those without, (3) that second generation Americans should have higher cancer rates than first or third generation Americans, (4) that cancer rates in a country at war should go down if the country is united and up if the country is disrupted, and (5) that paranoid schizophrenics should have high cancer rates while other schizophrenics should have low cancer rates. All of these hypotheses, generated largely on the idea that cancer rates should be strongly affected by the degree to which an individual can feel an attachment to some social group, are borne out by the data provided in the paper. Obviously some of the hypotheses are at variance with the accepted risk factors for breast cancer mentioned earlier in this chapter. Others, such as the cancer rates for schizophrenics, are not universally accepted (Perrin and Pierce, 1959; Fox, 1978) but are supported by various studies (Scheflen, 1951; Achterberg, Collerain and Craig, 1978), though there are many explanations besides strength of object cathexes that could be advanced.

Fisher and Cleveland (1956) analyzed Rorschach records of 89 patients with either 'interior' (largely cervical) or 'exterior' (largely breast) cancers and found higher barrier and lower penetration-of-boundary scores, again somewhat subjective objective measures, in the latter. Their control group, 28 patients who had had colostomies for colon cancer, did not differ from the interior group. The authors' hypothesis was that this supported the view that personality played a role in determining the location of development of a cancer in a directly symbolic fashion.

Based on an analysis of Rorschach records of 30 cancer patients, Klopfer (1957) felt that people with slow-growing cancer had a general attitude of unconcern while those with fast-growing cancer tried very hard to be good and loyal. He postulated that the patients with fast-growing cancers had so much vital energy tied up in defense of the ego that they did not have enough to defend against cancer.

LeShan and Reznikoff (1960), in another study relating loss of an important relationship in childhood to some specific statistic through a chain of inference oblivious to the many other possible intervening variables, studied the families of 200 cancer patients and found, as they had predicted, that cancer patients had a shorter period of being a youngest child than did their siblings.

Further elaboration of LeShan's idea of the basic psychological make-up of cancer patients was provided in 1961 when, based on a sample size now greater than 300 patients, he added despair to the constellation of experiences of the cancer patient. He described this as a feeling of absolute aloneness and no hope that there is any way that this will change. He concluded that this was an outgrowth of the early experiences he had previously noted. This was a descriptive paper and made no effort to provide numerical data.

Shrifte (1962) reported an analysis of Rorschachs on 22 indigent women with cervical cancer, divided into a good and bad prognosis group two years after testing. An initial hypothesis that the bad prognosis group would show 'massive, unresolved, unpleasant feeling tension' was not borne out at all and was abandoned, and based on an analysis once the groups were known, a second hypothesis was proposed: that the bad prognosis group showed a higher ratio of expenditure responses to consumption responses than the good prognosis group (though the actual ratio used would appear from the paper to only be concerned with expenditure). Consumption was judged from responses utilizing form, color and shading; expenditure was judged by movement responses. This hypothesis was tested on two other groups, men with malignancies and women with good prognoses), and in both cases statistical validation was found. The author suggests that bad prognosis individuals are those who are 'victims of undischarged, dammed up, wasted, unused vitality' at the same time that they have the 'potential of draining themselves' because they are unable to take in vitality.

Renneker *et al.* (1963) described a phenomenologic survey of the developmental histories and psychotherapy for five women with breast cancer. They noted a general pattern of oral-dependent deprivation by the patients' mothers, identification with those masochistic mothers, and subsequent depression at the loss of an important object. Their hypothesis was that this depression lowered host resistance, probably in some way related to hormone levels, a harbinger of the interest that was developing in finding a biological substrate to the possible relationships of stress and cancer.

Following up on a Swedish study that had suggested that women who develop cancer are more likely to be substable (a personality factor akin to extraversion), Coppen and Metcalfe (1963) studied 47 women with cancer and 94 age-matched controls, some with other illnesses and others disease-free, with the Maudsley Personality Inventory. Cancer patients, particularly breast cancer patients, had significantly higher extraversion scores, a finding particularly noteworthy because it is so seemingly antithetical to most of what had been proposed about cancer patients before (and what was to be proposed).

Booth (1965), writing from a more psychoanalytic approach, presented a comparison of Rorschach responses from cancer patients and tuberculosis patients and reached just an opposite conclusion. He described cancer patients as characterized by an anal attitude towards objects, striving to retain control in relationships and to avoid emotional involvement, and he felt it was no accident that Freud was a cancer patient himself. He also advocated more attention to the psychological needs of cancer patients, even if it was not to prolong their lives.

Interest in this area was now keen enough that in 1965 a conference entitled 'Psychophysiological Aspects of Cancer' was held by the New York Academy of Sciences and the papers published in their *Annals* the next year. Muslin, Gyarfas and Pieper (1966) discussed a study of women with breast cancer compared with women with benign breast lesions, who were given questionnaires pertaining to separation experiences prior to their breast biopsies. After forming two matched groups with respect to race, age, marital status and socioeconomic class, they found no support for increases in early or recent separations in the malignant group. This remained true when comparing data obtained from interviews with the patients. Bahnson and Bahnson (1966) reported results of using various projective methods, including interviews, structured questionnaires, Rorschach tests and the Bahnson Rhythmical Apperception Test (where subjects were asked to describe neutral auditory stimuli with emotionally meaningful words), to assess ego defenses in cancer patients and some controls. They found a consistent pattern of denying and repressing conflicting emotions, particularly hostility and guilt. Hagnell (1966) (amplifying the study that had triggered the Coppen and Metcalfe study) reported that in a ten-year prospective study of 2250 persons in a selected area in Sweden, it was found that there was a statistically significantly higher number of cases of cancer in substable women, but not in substable men. This was among the first prospective studies in this area. Another significant aspect of the conference was the extent to which neuroendocrinologic ideas were being developed, a sign of the preeminence that biologic formulations were assuming over more strictly psychosomatic ones; Grinker (1966), addressing the latter view, stated, 'we have no right to assert at this time that psychological factors are significant in locating the site of cancer'.

In 1967, Goldfarb, Driesen and Cole reported on three cases of women with breast cancer and depression who were given ECT and chemotherapy and experienced 'positive cancerocidal effects', apparently beyond what the authors thought chemotherapy alone would produce. The possible explanations they suggested for this were lowering of free fatty acid levels, formation of an antibody-like substance, stimulation of the CNS, a cancer-inhibiting electromagnetic field, and a renewed ability to defend against the cancer due to resolution of the depression.

Stavraky (1968) tested 204 patients with cancer, administering the MMPI and a test called the Differential Diagnostic Technique (DDT), designed to reveal basic personality characteristics. The quartiles with the least and most favorable outcomes (excepting that some of the early breast and cervical cancer patients were excluded; they apparently were included among the average outcome control group) were compared. The DDT indicated tendencies for all cancer patients to show loss of control of emotions and hostility compared to the normals reported for the test. In addition, the most favorable outcome group showed significantly fewer normal values and significantly more hostility without loss of emotional control than their stage-matched control group (hostility or dependency were the two poles of the scale). The group with the least favorable outcome was not decidedly different on any tests. An attempt to replicate Blumberg's results with the MMPI revealed no difference between any of the groups.

In 1968, a Second Conference On Psychophysiological Aspects Of Cancer was held by the New York Academy of Sciences and published in 1969. Bahnson (1969) reported the results of a parent–child questionnaire that indicated that cancer patients retrospectively perceive their parents as having been more neglecting than normal controls. In another paper, Bahnson and Bahnson (1969) elaborated on the Bahnson Rhythmical Apperception Test reported three years earlier, noting that they had tested 30 men with cancer, 64 men without disease, 33 men with a first myocardial infarction and 26 men with other illnesses. Data analysis (using an elaborately determined and somewhat difficult formula) revealed that, as predicted, the cancer patients projected less anxiety, depression, hostility or dominance than either of the other groups. They projected as much guilt as the other ill subjects, though still less than the normals. This was interpreted as indicating that cancer patients project fewer unpleasant emotions into the environment and therefore repress more of them. Katz *et al.* (1969, 1970) described a study of 32 women who had entered a hospital for breast biopsy and whose hormone levels and psychological disruption were measured, the latter by assessment of interviews. Those women who appeared to have more defensive failing had higher hydrocortisone production rates, but there were no psychological differences (in terms of affective distress, disruption of ego functions or impairment of defensive reserve) or differences in androgen levels found between those women whose tumor proved to be malignant and those where it was proved to be benign. In contrast to the previous conference, there were more theoretical papers presented, and these focussed not only on the neuroendocrinologic aspects of the problem but on the immunologic aspects, the idea that psychophysiologically impaired immunity could lead to cancer.

Achte and Vauhkonen (1979) described a study done in Finland of 100 cancer patients along various psychological parameters. They culled out two subgroups with extremes of survival and compared the two, finding that those who died sooner tended to have not asked about the nature of their illness, to be more depressed and anxious, to be more aggressive and to be more hopeless. They also tended to have more advanced disease. No statistical analysis was done. In the same volume, Viitamaki (1970) reported on a battery of psychological tests given to the same patients to see if any variables correlated with the malignity stage of the cancer at detection and the survival time of the patients after detection (in both of these studies, it appears that absolute survival time, not that relative to others with the same disease, was used). He found no significant correlations with stage of cancer, but noted that, out of 50 variables, a combination of three psychiatric and eight psychological variables, which seemed to relate to more ego strength, less anxiety, less depression, more knowledge of condition and (apparently, though it is hard to tell from how the data are presented) less aggression, was significantly correlated with longer survival times.

A study of 352 women with breast cancer and 670 women with other cancers and non-cancerous diseases was reported by Snell and Graham (1971) exploring whether the former would report more stressful events having occurred in the five years prior to their diagnosis. They found no such difference, but suggested that if one had been found, its genesis would probably have been endocrinologic.

Prospective investigation of this question was again introduced with the reporting of the Johns Hopkins Precursors Study, through which 1337 medical students at Johns Hopkins from 1948 to 1964 were given a series of psychological tests when medically well and were then followed to monitor correlations between those results and the development of several diseases, one of which was cancer. In a series of papers (Thomas and Greenstreet, 1973; Thomas and Duszynski, 1974; Thomas, 1976; Thomas, Duszynski and Shaffer, 1979; Duszynski, Shaffer and Thomas, 1981) these results were reported. They indicated that those who developed cancer had habits of nervous tension (depression, anger and anxiety from a Habits of Nervous Tension questionnaire) similar to those of normals, but reported significantly less closeness to parents, less demonstrative parents and less matriarchal dominance than others (on a Family Attitude questionnaire). They also noted a multiple discriminant analysis of Rorschach and psychobiological variable that could reasonably separate out the cancer group, but cautioned about the difficulty of drawing major conclusions from this. What traits a typical cancer-prone person would have on the basis of this analysis was not explicated. In a further effort to confirm or refute previously reported findings, they analyzed the data to see whether subjects who developed cancer had more parental deaths, more parental divorces, more sibling deaths or less time spent as a youngest child than healthy subjects. Although there were trends towards three of these hypotheses being statistically significant, none was. Even after combining the total number of these traumatic events, although there was a numerical trend for major cancer>skin cancer>benign tumor>healthy control, it was not statistically significant. Addressing why their results differed from those of some previous studies, they pointed out that, because they had a relatively small (30) number of subjects with major cancer, they might not have had enough patients to find correlations of small magnitude, but also noted that this, being a confirmatory study, could avoid some methodologic pitfalls that might have affected the exploratory research done previously.

Another non-confirmatory study was presented by Schonfield (1975), who interviewed 112 women on the day prior to a breast biopsy and gave them selected MMPI scales (Lie, Depression and Well-Being), a Holmes and Rahe Schedule of Recent Experiences and an IPAT (a scale for measuring covert and overt anxiety). None of these results was found to be significantly correlated with the eventual finding of a malignant tumor at the 0.05 significance level (although the article reported two correlations at the 0.10 level: higher covert anxiety and Lie scale scores in women under 42 with malignant disease). In fact, the women with benign tumors had a significantly higher number of life change units.

In a similar vein, Greer and Morris (1975, 1978) interviewed and administered a series of psychological questionnaires to 160 women who were being admitted to a hospital for breast biopsy. The women with benign and malignant disease were similar with respect to marital state, social class, incidence of psychiatric disorders, social adjustment, sexual adjustment (a nonsignificant trend for the women with cancer to be less so was noted), verbal intelligence, hostility (by a Hostility questionnaire), extraversion, neuroticism, reported style of reacting to stress, occurrence of stressful life events, loss of a loved one and L(ie) scale scores on the Eysenck Personality Inventory. The women with cancer were as a group significantly older. Even after adjustment for age, they showed more abnormal release of anger (either expressing very little or very much), and, in certain age groups, other emotions as well. Which ones were not specified.

In a follow-up study, the same group of women was investigated with respect to immunoglobulin levels (Pettingale, Greer and Tee, 1977). In general, women who were classified as extreme suppressors of anger had higher levels of IgA. IgG, IgM and IgE levels were not disparate. The authors suggested that this was a psychobiological link that might play some part in the pathogenesis of breast cancer since it had already been shown that extreme suppressors of anger were more likely to develop breast cancer. Why women who were extreme expressors of anger should develop breast cancer more was not explained. As in the previous report, there were no normal controls. No correlation with cancer prognosis was attempted, although, if this is any indication of mortality, two year follow-ups were available for a smaller percentage of the normal expressors than for the two extreme groups.

The first reported study concerning variables affecting the prognosis of already diagnosed cancer patients was that of Weisman and Worden (1975). They gathered psychosocial information about 46 terminal or preterminal cancer patients and coded it on their Terminality/Lethality Index, which included demographic data and attitudes about illness and death. Using a survival quotient developed to estimate relative survival across several types of cancer, they found that by one analysis a group of eight variables was significantly correlated with longer survival times. Socioeconomic class and variables they called rising resentment, terminal apathy and terminal cooperation were positively correlated; early separation, poor social relationships, death wish and acceptance of death were negatively correlated. (In a zero order correlation it appears that early separation is not significantly correlated, but maternal suicide is; the other correlations remain intact.) They concluded that patients with longer survival times seemed to be those who had good relationships with others, had parents who were less absent in their childhood, and were able to ask others for support. They might have a tendency to deny the seriousness of their illness and might express some resentment about their condition, but they did not tend to be depressed. This was the first study to suggest that a general pattern of social support was of positive value in cancer as opposed to some specific life history event or personality style.

A different approach to the problem was undertaken by Voth (1976), who reported on two samples of cancer patients tested for autokinesis, the perceived motion of a pinpoint of light in total darkness, and field-dependence (using the embedded figures test). A first sample comprised 31 subjects from another study who some time after being tested developed cancer; a second sample comprised 24 women with breast cancer. Compared with controls, though it is not clear how closely controls were matched for demographic and other variables, both cancer groups showed less autokinesis and more field-dependence. The authors noted that in previous studies these findings had been associated with a higher tendency to use repression and to become depressed.

Forty-four men with cancer and a similar number of matched non-cancer controls were given structured interviews by Smith and Sebastian (1976). The patients were rated as to overall intensity and duration of emotionally critical incidents over their lifetimes and it was found that the cancer patients had a dramatically higher number and intensity of such incidents. No statistical analysis is presented.

Watson and Schuld (1977) published a semiprospective study of 50 patients from mid-Western VA hospitals who had been given MMPIs at least two years prior to the diagnosis of benign or malignant neoplasms and 50 age-matched controls. Initially the malignant and benign groups both showed significantly higher F(ake) or L(ie) scales, so the controls were rematched to exclude F and L variability. When this was done, there were no significant differences among the three groups on MMPI scores or psychiatric diagnosis. The authors concluded that this research offered 'no support for the psychogenic theories of neoplastic growth'. What is to be made of the fact that there was a significant difference immediately evident and that this was then eliminated for data analysis is not addressed.

Studying the hospital records of all women admitted to a large university hospital over a ten-year period who were found to have breast cancer or another cancer, Overall (1978) found no difference in the frequency of prior psychiatric treatment between the two groups. This was intended as an investigation of whether psychotropic medications (particularly neuroleptics, which raise prolactin levels) would increase the risk of breast cancer, but it also addresses to some extent whether women with breast cancer exhibit any particular psychological vulnerabilities.

To compare the relative strengths of proposed psychological factors in different age groups, Becker (1979) interviewed 49 women with breast cancer. He found that those below 50 years of age described a significantly higher number of separations from parents before age fourteen, a less positive family atmosphere, more marital difficulties, less sexual responsiveness, more negative attitudes towards children, more psychosomatic symptoms, more problems with pregnancy and breastfeeding and more recent losses of a partner. Although there were no other control groups, this was interpreted to support previous hypotheses about the psychological precursors to cancer, an 'Amazon complex' where women assumed a combative attitude and took on men's roles, often in a self-destructive way. Becker further suggested that this took its toll through weakening the immune system and that it was not as evident in older women because they were more subject to other carcinogenic factors and, in addition, experienced a general weakening of the immune system because of age.

Derogatis, Abeloff and Melisaratos (1979) studied 35 women with metastatic breast cancer, interviewing them and administering several self-report and objective instruments. Based on their subsequent length of survival (one year being the cutoff), they divided the patients into two groups and found that the short-term survivors reported significantly less hostility, depression and guilt, in fact general distress, on the self-report scales and significantly more positive attitudes towards their illness and physicians on the externally rated scales. The only significant difference between the two groups medically was that the short-term survival group had greater exposure to chemotherapy. They suggested that these results were the result of immunologic or endocrine influences.

In a study of 6928 randomly selected California adults who were followed for nine-year mortality, Berkman and Syme (1979) found that increased mortality was significantly correlated with fewer social and community ties. For the most and least isolated groups, the mortality rates differed by a factor greater than two. This was so even after taking into account the presence of preexisting physical illness, socioeconomic status, smoking, obesity, alcohol use, physical activity and utilization of health services. Although no data are mentioned in the body of the paper, the authors note that this increased mortality was also evident in considering specific causes of death, including cancer. Several mechanisms by which this might be explained are proposed, including psychological responses that reduce coping abilities and physiologic (e.g. nervous, hormonal or immunologic) changes that increase susceptibility to disease.

Greer, Morris and Pettingale (1979) studied 69 consecutive early stage breast cancer patients who were treated with simple mastectomy with clinical and psychological assessments and followed them for five years. Their initial psychological response to cancer was categorized using patients' statements and accompanying mood as (1) denial, (2) fighting spirit, (3) stoic acceptance or (4) helplessness/hopelessness. The latter two responses were significantly associated with poorer outcome after five years, as was being unmarried or having poor marital relationships. Most other variables, including habitual reaction to stressful events, expression/suppression of anger, depression, hostility, sexual adjustment, interpersonal relationships, extraversion and verbal intelligence, were not associated with poor outcome. Apparently response to cancer was considered state-specific and not indicative of a personality trait. These authors, too, felt that neuroendocrine or immunologic explanations were most likely. In a follow-up report (Pettingale *et al.*, 1985) at ten years, this association between response and outcome was still evident, as was the lack of other associations.

MMPI profiles obtained at least one year before diagnosis on 75 veterans with cancer and 125 without were analyzed by Dattore, Shontz and Coyne (1980). They found a linear discriminant function, made up mostly of the Repression–Sensitization, Depression and Denial of Hysteria scales, that significantly distinguished between the two groups. The cancer group was lower on all three scales, indicating more tendency to use repression, less depression and more introspection. This was based on samples that had a significant difference in mean age (cancer—64 years, non-cancer—54 years), and although certain other analyses were done to demonstrate how that did not affect the final result, the discriminant function itself was not recalculated using groups comparable in age. The authors also point out that while the discrimination was significant, it was not of great magnitude, and actual attempts to distinguish cancer-prone patients would yield a low rate of correct classifications. The results were interpreted as supportive of previous theories of psychological cancer-proneness.

On the other hand, Shekelle *et al.* (1981) administered MMPIs to 2107 middle-aged male Western Electric employees and followed them for 17 years. Those men with a high depression score had double the risk of death from cancer, unaffected by age, smoking, alcohol use, family history of cancer or occupation. They suggest immunologic effects of depression as a tentative explanation for this.

Reporting on 123 patients seen at a cancer counseling center in Texas, Simonton and Matthews-Simonton (1981) reported that median survival times for patients with advanced breast, bowel and lung cancer undergoing psychotherapy were markedly longer than the national median survival times for those diseases. No statistical analysis was done. Therapy included 're-deciding early-life decisions, improving emotional outlets . . ., goal-setting . . ., identifying stress, and identifying secondary gains of illness'. Relaxation and mental imagery exercises were also considered key. They regarded this as a preliminary study, but one which supported the idea that counseling can improve the quality and length of life of cancer patients.

Following up on their previous studies, Morris *et al.* (1981) reported on a study of 50 women admitted for breast biopsy. They were interviewed and given the Eysenck Personality Questionnaire and an anxiety inventory. The women were then rated on an expression of anger scale developed by the authors (scores ranged from 1—'does not admit to feeling anger ever since 21', to 6—'loses control in anger at least once a month in front of adults'). The seventeen women who had breast cancer (who, as in other studies, had a significantly higher mean age) were found to have significantly lower expression of anger scores than the 33 with benign disease. When only compared with women of similar age, this finding was 'marginally significant' for women between the ages of 40 and 49. In this last group of women, cancer patients had a significantly lower N(euroticism) score on the Eysenck without a statistically increased L(ie) score, although the authors note a 'tendency' for these women to have high L scores. These results were interpreted to suggest that young women with breast cancer tend to be telling the truth when they say that they express anger less freely than those with benign disease, i.e. to lie behaviorally about the anger that they feel. An alternative hypothesis, it seems, would have been that those women lie when they say they express anger less freely.

The mortality in 4032 white widowed Marylanders during a ten-year period (Helsing and Szklo, 1981; Helsing, Comstock and Szklo, 1982) was compared with that of a similar number of married matched controls. Widowed men showed a significantly greater mortality, but women showed no difference. There was no significant difference in the mortality from cancer for any of the groups; the authors conclude that the increased mortality of the widowed men is 'remarkably non-specific as to its causes'.

Funch and Marshall (1983) reported a 20-year follow-up study of 208 white women with breast cancer who had been evaluated at diagnosis regarding degree of social support and objective (e.g. death in household) and subjective (e.g. tired feelings) stress in the five years preceding diagnosis. They reported that lower total stress and more organizational involvement were significantly associated with longer survival. Stage, however, was by far the best predictor of survival, better actually than a combination of stage, stress and social support for the entire sample. A model using the above three factors in the sample excluding those age 46–60 (apparently because they seemed to show less of the desired correlation with those factors) was better than one using stage alone, but still only predicted 13 per cent of the total variance, suggesting 'that a number of other factors are also involved in survival'.

Studying a 1 per cent sample of the population of England and Wales for cancer incidence and mortality following widowhood, Jones, Goldblatt and Leon (1984) found that five-year follow-up suggested only a very slight increase in mortality and not one that was statistically significant. There was a greater, though still not significant, indication that mortality from other causes was increased.

Self-perceptions of 222 women, about evenly divided as to having breast cancer, benign breast disease and no disease, were investigated with five questionnaires (Jansen and Muenz, 1984). Because the groups differed significantly on four of seven demographic variables, an analysis of covariance was used to analyze the data. There were significant differences on five of the 30 psychological scales. These suggested that healthy women will describe themselves as calm, outgoing and expressive of anger; women with fibrocystic disease will describe themselves as tense, outgoing and expressive of anger; and women with breast cancer will describe themselves as calm, unassertive and unexpressive of anger.

Priestman, Priestman and Bradshaw (1985), noting the continued interest in life stresses and the development of cancer, reported on three groups of 100 women each (with breast cancer, benign breast disease, and no disease) who were questioned regarding life stresses over the three years preceding diagnosis and given the Eysenck Personality Inventory (EPI). The control women had significantly higher life stress scores, while the benign and malignant groups showed no difference on the EPI. The authors, after reviewing previous negative studies, concluded that antecedent life stresses still did not predispose to breast cancer.

A study of both immunologic and behavioral associations with breast cancer prognosis was reported by Levy *et al.* (1985). Seventy-five women with breast cancer were interviewed and rated on the Global Adjustment to Illness Scale, given the Symptom Checklist-90 and Profile of Mood States, and assayed for natural killer (NK) cell (a cytotoxic lymphocyte) activity. Correlations were found between higher NK activity and fewer positive nodes, and between lower NK activity and ratings of being well adjusted, fatigued and unsupported socially. Correlations were not found between self-reported distress and cancer status (number of positive axillary nodes), observer-reported adjustment and cancer status, or perception of social support and cancer status. In addition, and significantly for the question of interpretation of what self-report scales really reflect, no correlation was found between self-reported adjustment and observer-reported adjustment. These results were proposed to support the idea that behavior and cancer risk are related and that they are related through an immunologic mechanism.

In a sample of 6928 Californians who were followed from 1965 to 1982 (reported by Bower, 1986), Reynolds and Kaplan found after controlling for age, smoking, alcohol, initial physical health and income that women (but not men) with fewer social contacts were more likely to die from cancer, the risk being fivefold for hormone-dependent cancers and threefold for cancer as a whole. Even a feeling of social isolation without decreased social contacts was associated with a higher risk. Depression by itself was not.

In yet another study of loss and breast cancer, Ewertz (1986) reported that, comparing 1782 Danish women with breast cancer and 1738 controls, there was no significant association between widowhood (of any duration) and risk of breast cancer.

THE LITERATURE AS A WHOLE

What is to be made of this wealth of studies? Perhaps most obvious is that there are results to contradict most any of the other reported results. Breast cancer or cancer patients generally may have increased expression of anger, decreased expression of anger, normal expression of anger, more recent life stresses, fewer recent life stresses. Of course, as has been pointed out, both in the introduction and in several of the papers, breast cancer is a complex disease with many known risk factors, a fact which some authors do not seem to take into account in their zeal to demonstrate the importance of the psyche. It is no surprise, therefore, that different groups of patients, perhaps differing in ways that are not even yet quantifiable by present methods, should present with different psychological characteristics. If different subgroups of cancer patients did in fact respond to different degrees to different types of psychological variables, large general studies would only detect minimal and possibly contradictory influences, the more general the study the worse.

Another observation, especially considering the potential methodologic problems noted earlier, is the number of such problems in the studies: by and large they are retrospective, some use measurement tools of limited validation, and even widely accepted tools, for example the Rorschach or Eysenck Personality Inventory, may be questioned as to proper method of interpretation. Self-report measures are taken to be true reflections of external behaviors of patients, even though the same patients are noted to try to present a good front on test-taking.

One may get the impression that at least some of the studies were interpreted with an eye to supporting preformed opinions: groups of patients are excluded because they do not seem to fit expectations, the one potentially positive finding is highlighted while other negative findings are mentioned in passing, or large-scale data manipulations are described, the validity of which is not assessable by the non-statisticswise reader (one wonders, for example, what the results of other equally plausible groupings of patients would be in those studies where certain age groups or stress types are combined for ease of comparison). Sometimes it seems the cancer patient cannot win—a high MMPI D score indicates that the patient is depressed, a low MMPI D score indicates that she is depressed but repressing or denying it. And, if low scores of a measured variable indicate that the variable is more repressed, the question still remains how much of the repressed variable cancer patients have relative to normals and whether that is important.

There are questions, too, about the interpretation of the terminology that is used in trying to decide if studies have similar or contradictory results. Is one author's 'repression' the same as another author's 'denial', another author's 'suppression' or even the same as another author's 'repression'? Is denial of the seriousness of illness different from repression of unpleasant emotions? And does suppression of anger mean not losing control of anger or not expressing it outwardly in any form?

One must clearly, then, take a panoramic view of the data presented. Table 1 is a rough abstraction of the results reported in the studies discussed above. Given the disparate nature of the way that results were reported and interpreted, it is of course impossible to make precise classifications, but the data are sorted as well as possible. It is also important to remember that, since many of the studies were written with an eye to reporting positive results, there may be some negative results that are not caught in the net of summary statements.

One sees that, despite the limitations described, there may be evidence for psychological factors affecting the development and growth of breast cancer, but only insofar as they affect cancer generally, no factors having been consistently found specifically referable to breast cancer.

The loss of a significant relationship is not one of these. There have been multiple studies discounting such an association, and, as the natural history of at least breast cancer suggests, this would be expected to be so. The studies having to do with conflicts over sexuality were done early, in the era of psychosomatic specificity, and no more recent studies have been done to verify or refute those observations.

However, studies of the development of cancer do suggest that a decreased outward expression of 'negative' emotions is associated with negative outcome. Studies of the course of cancer once diagnosed suggest the same. That the answers to these two independently considered questions are the same and that these two questions turn out on further consideration likely to be the same question provides even more support for the answers having some truth.

Table 1

Proposed factor	Number of studies	
	Positive	Negative
Loss of important relationship/increased life stress	7	9
Emotional calm/repression	16	4
Disturbed upbringing	9	1
Conflicts over sexuality	3	0
Despair/depression	6	4
Extraversion	2	2
Hostility	4	3
Loss of emotional control	2	1
Poor social supports	4	0

Although not as well studied, there are indications from a variety of approaches—one of the few prospective studies, retrospective studies and clinical impressions—that the amount of social support, in growing up and in adult life, is correlated with cancer morbidity and mortality. Whether this social isolation is a manifestation of other psychological variables, such as personality traits, is left unanswered, though it would seem likely. A potentially associated condition, something variously called 'hopelessness' or 'despair', is not overwhelmingly supported overall, but the analysis of this is complicated by the differentiation of hopelessness from depression with its myriad meanings (e.g. clinical depression, high MMPI D scale scores).

Especially with regard to the last condition, additional evidence to support the validity of that psychological influence on neoplasm comes in the form of case reports of spontaneous regressions of cancer. An occurrence of such rarity (about one in 100 000 cases) that it is difficult to investigate in any controlled fashion, spontaneous regression of cancer is nevertheless an accepted phenomenon (Stoll, 1979), and anecdotal reports frequently link its development to a condition of hope or belief in the possibility of improvement. A particularly striking example mentioned by Klopfer (1957) concerns a man with generalized lymphosarcoma whose condition, thought to be preterminal, remitted almost totally for two months while he was receiving injections of Krebiozen, an experimental drug he thought would cure him. After learning from the news that the drug was probably useless, he relapsed, only to recover for another two months when he was given water injections that he was told were a refined preparation of the same drug. Several days after a nationwide announcement that Krebiozen was definitely worthless, the patient relapsed and died.

Other ancillary data supporting the influence of stress on cancer come from a variety of animal studies that show increased stress promoting the development and growth of cancer (e.g. Andervont, 1944; Reznikoff and Martin, 1957; Sklar and Anisman, 1979). However, even in this potentially more controllable research area, variables are so numerous that, after a review of the literature, Peters and Mason (1979) can conclude, 'It is apparent from the data reviewed that experimental support can be found for essentially any view concerning the influence of stress on neoplasia'. They nevertheless go on to say that 'certain experimental observations are consistent enough to warrant consideration of the mechanisms involved to see whether these might be operative in man'. Although they were not examined here, these studies certainly give added credence to the likelihood of some similar relationship in man.

In summary, there are indications that certain psychological factors can influence the development and growth of breast cancer. These same factors seem to be operative in cancer as whole. However, these influences have not yet been definitively proven. Further, several studies note that the magnitude of this influence may be small, at least as it applies to a population of patients. It may be that in certain individuals there is a much larger influence, but with the heterogeneous nature of any patient sample this cannot be demonstrated. It will take more extensive and more carefully constructed research to validate these possibilities if scientific proof is sought.

POSSIBLE ETIOLOGIC MECHANISMS

The fascinating question still remains, if the above hypotheses are indeed true, how do those psychological factors exert their influence?

Many suggestions have been made over the years, but recently two schools of thought have been preeminent: (1) psychological factors operate through affecting the immune system or (2) they operate through affecting the endocrine system (which could also work through affecting the immune system). Besides appearing in the scientific literature, these are the theories the general reader finds in the books that inform him how patients can psychologically affect their cancers (LeShan, 1977; Simonton, Matthews-Simonton and Creighton, 1978).

The immune hypothesis is based on the theory of immune surveillance, an idea proposed by Thomas and Burnet that attracted wide interest in the 1970s. According to that theory, neoplastic cells are regularly formed in the body, but the immune system, through killer lymphocytes and possibly other immunologic mechanisms, is regularly eliminating them as they form. If this immune surveillance is impaired, the theory goes, more neoplastic cells escape destruction, and the risk for development of cancer is greater.

Many articles have been written advocating this position, though few actually examine the merits of the theory, perhaps because it is an appealing one to accept. The evidence for immune surveillance itself is really beyond the scope of this chapter, but it includes indications, largely from animal models, that natural killer (NK) cells have cytotoxic activity against primary tumor and metastatic cells and observations that populations (animal or human) with defects in NK activity have increased rates of certain neoplasms. In addition there have been reports that patients with advanced cancer have decreased NK activity, though no conclusions can be drawn regarding the direction of causality of this observation. The evidence that links immune surveillance to psychological risk factors in cancer consists of studies indicating impaired immune responses in animals and humans in varying stressful situations (for fuller reviews, see Locke *et al.*, 1984; Levy, 1985); it appears that little work has been done on immunologic activity and long-term psychological factors like personality traits.

Unfortunately the theory of immune surveillance has been under attack since early in its ascendancy (e.g. Moeller and Moeller, 1975), and there is strong support in present-day oncologic thinking (e.g. Bast, 1985) for the position that, while immune surveillance does exist, it is of much less importance than has been thought in the past, and it may not even be operative in all types of cancer. After an extensive review, Stutman (1983) concluded that immunological surveillance 'remains as a limited event that may apply to a limited number of tumors, and which in some cases can be interpreted by alternative hypotheses'. Among the strongest evidence for the view that immunosurveillance has limited applicability is that found in the study of cancer in immunosuppressed humans, both congenital and acquired. Blattner and Hoover (1985) note that though humans with immune deficits, whether from congenital immunodeficiency, drug-induced immunodeficiency or other altered immunity states including AIDS, do have higher rates of malignancy, these higher rates are only for certain specific types of cancer, notably lymphoreticular neoplasms and soft-tissue sarcomas. They do not include many other common cancers, such as breast. Thus, in the population in the best position to demonstrate the true effect of impaired immunity on the development of cancer, there is 'no general diathesis of malignancy'.

What effect can one expect if stress (or, being generous, personality) does lead to impaired immunity? Even supporters of the theory report that 'the differences we have observed (in a study on the effects of life stresses on natural killer cell activity) are quite small and of uncertain clinical significance' (Locke *et al.*, 1984). Immune surveillance alone appears to be an incomplete explanation of whatever association there is between psyche and cancer.

The endocrinologic theory notes that psychological stress changes levels of multiple hormones and suggests that these changes can foster tumor growth (Stoll, 1985). Some hormones (e.g. adrenocortical steroids) might exert their effect through altering immune function (though, as we have seen, that is a rather unfortunate avenue to invoke); some might have more or less direct effects on the tumor. To take the case of breast cancer, it is well accepted that, as earlier noted, certain hormonal levels are clearly of some influence in the process of the disease.

Nevertheless, problems abound in trying to clarify the situation in even such a clearly hormone-dependent cancer as breast carcinoma. The important hormones seem to be estrogens, androgens and prolactin. The effects of stress on these hormones vary markedly in humans. Stress may produce increased, decreased or unaffected estrogen levels (Rakoff, 1962). Stress may produce increased, decreased, or unaffected androgen levels (Lobo *et al.*, 1983; Rose *et al.*, 1969; Parker *et al.*, 1985). Only prolactin seems to regularly change in one direction with stress: up (Mason, 1975), which is in fact the direction that would correlate with increased cancer. But the importance of prolactin in breast cancer is still unclear (Miller and Bulbrook, 1980) and the elevations in prolactin may only be intermittent (Harrison, O'Moore and O'Moore, 1986), also clouding the prediction of possible effects.

It has become increasingly clear that, while there are undeniably endocrine effects of psychological stressors, what effects are produced show marked intra-individual variation, depending on the stressor, how it is perceived and the personality traits and defensive functioning of the person experiencing the stress. Arnetz and Fjellner (1986) stressed 20 subjects with a colour–word conflict test and noted that endocrine changes ranged from positive to negative on all the variables measured (adrenaline, noradrenaline, cortisol, growth hormone, prolactin, progesterone and glucose). They found correlations of some of these changes with personality variables and concluded that 'psychosocial and cortical processes will intervene and are likely to influence neuroendocrine stress reactions strongly'.

This does not mean that psychoendocrine factors could not be operative in cancer, but it does mean that different ones might only be operative in certain groups of patients and that any attempt to find evidence of their operation in an unselected group of patients would likely be confounded. Furthermore not all cancers appear to be hormone-dependent, not even all breast cancers. If the endocrine theory (at least by itself) were correct, it would be surprising to find any positive results at all in the reported studies, when in fact there are a number of them.

What other possible factors are there? None has been as extensively investigated as the previous two, but several have been proposed. Among them are that stress predisposes to cancer through the mobilization of free fatty acids (Cardon and Mueller, 1966) or through the alteration of the body's response to tumor angiogenesis factor, since vascularization is essential to tumor or metastatic growth (Sklar and Anisman, 1981). Obviously, any biologic mechanism that either enhances or inhibits tumor growth, for example the hypothetical endogenous mitotic inhibitors called chalones (Houck and Attallah, 1975), could be a possible target for stress-induced alterations.

In general, the above theories suggest a bodywide sphere of influence of psychological effectors, but there are proponents of local effects being more important. Sklar and Anisman (1981), after a lengthy review of the subject, concluded that 'stress-induced alterations of tumor growth probably reflect local alterations of the microenvironment surrounding the tumor'. One piece of support for this, and a potentially important phenomenon in connection with the whole question at hand, is the one generally accepted case of psychological factors affecting the growth of a tumor: the influence of hypnosis on the common wart. Although the wart is a benign tumor, it is caused by one of the papovaviruses, most of which are potentially oncogenic (Nagington and Rook, 1979) and one strain of which, a human papillomavirus (HPV5), is definitely associated with squamous cell carcinoma in man (Pass, 1982). Standard dermatology textbooks (Domonkos and Arnold, 1982) acknowledge that warts can be cured by suggestion alone. One of the reported studies of the efficacy of hypnosis for treating warts (Sinclair-Gieben, 1959) used one half of the patient's body as the control for the other. Of the nine patients (out of fourteen) whose warts were cured on the treated side, only one of them also showed improvement in the warts on the other side (and this occurred six weeks after the treated side had responded). In this case, then, there is evidence to support the contention that psychological effects on tumor growth are local and not systemic.

The only major theory that would be consistent with the view that psychological effects on tumor growth are local is the theory of nervism (Corson, 1966): effects are produced through the mediation of the nervous system, which can alter such local conditions as the 'protective reactions of the connective tissue' (Kavetsy, Turkevich and Balitsky, 1966). Early reports (Cheatle, 1903, 1908; Cramer, cited in *British Medical Journal*, 1925; 1:1139) seemed to demonstrate that in animals, tumor growth could be affected by innervation of an area, whether natural or experimentally denervated, but there has been little work done on this in recent times. Indeed, there seems to have been little attention paid to this whole line of thought in recent times, largely it seems due to the immense interest in the immunologic theory. More investigation of this area would certainly be worthwhile.

Plainly, there is no one theory yet proposed that convincingly explains how psychological variables can influence the growth of cancer, if indeed they do. It would be more parsimonious to propose one mechanism for all cancers; still, nature is not always elegant. As has been noted earlier and as other reviewers of the question point out (Sklar and Anisman, 1981), it may be that the observed results are mediated through a combination of mechanisms, with different ones being of differing importance in different conditions. This becomes a much more difficult situation to sort out, but individual factors may still be detectable through more stringent control of study populations. Or it may be that the important mediating factor has not yet been found.

As a footnote, another idea regarding the way psychic factors may affect cancer that has appeared in one form or another for a long time is that some biological/psychic energy plays a role in maintaining health, and that when this is disturbed the appearance or growth of cancer results. A commonly held belief that there is a will to live and that loss of this, from belief in voodoo or resignation to mortality, among other things, can hasten death has been the subject of inquiry for many, including Freud, who touched on the subject with his speculations of life and death instincts (Freud, 1920), and, more recently, Stoll (1979) and Maguire (1979). Whatever one thinks of Reich's orgone energy or Kirlian photography (Ostrander and Shroeder, 1970; Krippner and Rubin, 1973), the concept of a life energy that is altered in illness states shows up so frequently, from so many different approaches (e.g. Riffenburgh (1969) produced a mathematical model that, starting with a consideration of the electrochemical properties of cells, derived a 'psychic kinetic drive force dimension' to explain the preneoplastic personality) and even across so many cultures that one must at least remain open to this idea.

FUTURE DIRECTIONS

The influence of psychological factors on the growth and development of breast cancer (and cancer in general) is still an unresolved question, and those who would maintain that there is conclusive evidence for or against it are perhaps influenced to take a premature stand by the emotional immensity of the topic. Nevertheless, there is sufficient research in the area to suggest that some relationship does exist, and that the factors that relate to breast cancer are no different than the factors that relate to other cancers.

It therefore follows that there may be psychological steps that some who have already developed cancer can take that will improve their prognoses. (It would follow, too, that there may be psychological steps that some could take to prevent the development of cancer, and this has in fact been proposed (Smith and Sebastian, 1976), but the multifactorial etiology of cancer makes this of more doubtful value, even if it is true.) Nevertheless, no satisfactory path by which these events might happen has yet been proposed. Clearly, what is warranted is more thought and more research; a definitive answer to either of these questions would be of great value. This is, unfortunately, more easily proposed than accomplished, for cancer is a complex disease, something which many researchers, in their enthusiasm, seem to overlook in trying to find the answers. Ultmann and Golomb (1983) note that 'Cancer is not one disease', and go on to point out that 'There are more than 100 clinically distinct forms of cancer, with differing biological behavior and clinical manifestations.' Of cancer, Pardee (1985) writes, 'Only the general properties of neoplasia and anaplasia appear evidently universal.' At whatever biological level psychological stresses are assumed to be operative, it would be well to keep this in mind in the construction of future studies.

A definitive answer will indeed be hard to ascertain. Prospective studies are difficult to produce, retrospective studies are inherently flawed, and any measurement tool, no matter how well constructed, may simply be unable to quantify the complexities of the actual issues involved, whether it be the subtleties of the psychological variables or the multiplicity of the biological influences. Complex constellations of psychological variables are not always amenable to numerically exact investigation, so continued consideration of the topic must include not only statistically validated results, but also the intuitive syntheses of those working in the field; as of yet, no more sensitive instrument for integrating emotional data has been discovered than the human observer.

It must be pointed out, too, that regardless of whether psychotherapy actually does prevent or modify the course of cancer, it can still aid the cancer patient in dealing with a serious and difficult illness. No solutions to the questions that this chapter has explored will change the fact that psychotherapy is a valuable adjunctive treatment for the cancer patient. But until a definitive answer is discovered as to the effects of emotions on cancer, psychological interventions should be regarded with an attitude open to the range of their effects, lest premature closure lead either to the loss of a valuable adjunctive treatment for those afflicted with cancer or to the promulgation of a false and inappropriately confident hope.

REFERENCES

Achte, K., and Vauhkonen, M. (1970). Psychic factors in Cancer, in *Cancer And Psyche, Monographs from the Psychiatric Clinic of Helsinki*, **1**, 3–44.

Achterberg, J., Collerain, I., and Craig, P. (1978). A possible relationship between cancer, mental retardation and mental disorders, *Soc. Sci. Med.*, **12**, 135.

Andersen, J. A., Nielsen, M., and Jensen, J. (1985). Essential histological findings in the female breast at autopsy, in *Early Breast Cancer—Histopathology, Diagnosis and Treatment* (Eds J. Zander and J. Baltzer), Springer-Verlag, New York, pp. 52–63.

Andervont, H. B. (1944). Influence of environment on mammary cancer in mice, *J. Nat. Cancer Inst.*, **4**, 579.

Arnetz, B. B., and Fjellner, B. (1986). Psychological predictors of neuroendocrine responses to mental stress, *J. Psychosom. Res.*, **30**, 297.

Bacon, C. L., Renneker, R., and Cutler, M. (1952). A psychosomatic survey of cancer of the breast, *Psychosom. Med.*, **14**, 453.

Bahnson, C. B. (1969). Psychophysiological complementarity in malignancies. *Ann. NY Acad. Sci.*, **164**, 319.

Bahnson, M. B., and Bahnson, C. B. (1969). Ego defenses in cancer patients, *Ann. NY Acad. Sci.*, **164**, 546.

Bahnson, C. B., and Bahnson, M. B. (1966). Role of the ego defenses: Denial and repression in the etiology of malignant neoplasm, *Ann. NY Acad. Sci.*, **125**, 856.

Bast, R. C. (1985). Principles of cancer biology: tumor immunology, in *Cancer— Principles & Practice of Oncology* (Eds V. T. DeVita, S. Hellman and S. Rosenberg), J. B. Lippincott, New York, pp. 125–150.

Becker, H. (1979). Psychodynamic aspects of breast cancer, *Psychother. Psychosom.*, **32**, 287.

Berkman, L. F., and Syme, S. L. (1979). Social networks, host resistance, and mortality: A nine-year follow-up study of Alameda County residents, *Am. J. Epidem.*, **109**, 186.

Bieliauskas, L. A., and Garron, D. C. (1982). Psychological depression and cancer, *Gen. Hosp. Psych.*, **4**, 187.

Blattner, W. A., and Hoover, R. N. (1985). Cancer in the immunosuppressed host, in *Cancer—Principles & Practice of Oncology* (Eds V. T. DeVita, S. Hellman and S. Rosenberg), J. B. Lippincott, New York, pp. 1999–2006.

Blumberg, E. M., West, P. M., and Ellis, F. W. (1954). A possible relationship between psychological factors and human cancer, *Psychosom. Med.*, **16**, 277.

Booth, G. (1965). Irrational complications of the cancer problem, *Am. J. Psychoan.*, **25**, 41.

Booth, G. (1969). General and organ-specific object relationships in cancer, *Ann. NY Acad. Sci.*, **164**, 568.

Bower, B. (1986). Social isolation: Female cancer risk? *Sci. News*, **129**, 166.

Butler, B. (1954). The use of hypnosis in the care of the cancer patient, *Cancer*, **7**, 1.

Cardon, P. V., and Mueller, P. S. (1966). A possible mechanism: Psychogenic fat mobilization, *Ann. NY Acad. Sci.*, **125**, 924.

Cheatle, G. L. (1903). Note upon a possible relationship between carcinoma and nerve or trophic areas, *Brit. Med. J.*, **1**, 904.

Cheatle, G. L. (1908). Observations on the spread and incidence of cancer, *Brit. Med. J.*, **1**, 437.

Coppen, A., and Metcalfe, M. (1963). Cancer and extraversion, *Brit. Med. J.*, **2**, 18.

Corson, S. A. (1966). Neuroendocrine and behavioral response patterns to psychologic stress and the problem of the target tissue in cerebrovisceral pathology, *Ann. NY Acad. Sci.*, **125**, 890.

Dattore, P. J., Shontz, F. C., and Coyne, L. (1980). Premorbid personality differentiation of cancer and noncancer groups: A test of the hypothesis of cancer proneness, *J. Consult. Clin. Psychol.*, **48**, 388.

Derogatis, L. R., Abeloff, M. D., and Melisaratos, N. (1979). Psychological coping mechanisms and survival time in metastatic breast cancer, *JAMA*, **242**, 1504.

Devitt, J. E. (1976). Clinical prediction of growth behaviour, in *Risk Factors in Breast Cancer* (Ed. B. Stoll), Year Book Medical Publ., Chicago.

Dew, R. A. (1981). Wilhelm Reich's cancer biopathy, in *Psychotherapeutic Treatment of Cancer Patients* (Ed. J. G. Goldberg), Free Press, New York, pp. 83–115.

Domonkos, A. N., and Arnold, H. L. (1982). *Andrews' Disease of the Skin*, 7th edn, W. B. Saunders, Philadelphia.

Donegan, W. L. (1979). Epidemiology of mammary cancer, in *Cancer Of The Breast* (Eds J. S. Spratt and W. L. Donegan), W. B. Saunders, Philadelphia, pp. 12–33.

Duszynski, K. R., Shaffer, J. W., and Thomas, C. B. (1981). Neoplasm and traumatic events in childhood, *Arch. Gen. Psych*, **38**, 327.

Ewertz, M. (1986). Bereavement and breast cancer, *Brit. J. Cancer*, **53**, 701.

Fisher, S., and Cleveland, S. E. (1956). Relationship of body image to site of cancer, *Psychosom. Med.*, **18**, 304.

Fournier, D., Hoeffken, W., Junkermann, H., Bauer, M., and Kuehn, W. (1985). Growth rate of primary mammary carcinoma and its metastases, in *Early Breast Cancer—Histopathology, Diagnosis and Treatment* (Eds J. Zander and J. Baltzer), Springer-Verlag, New York, pp. 73–86.

Fox, B. H. (1976). The psychosocial epidemiology of cancer, in *Cancer: The Behavioral Dimensions* (Eds J. W. Cullen, B. H. Fox and R. N. Isom), Raven Press, New York, pp. 11–22.

Fox, B. H. (1978). Cancer death risk in hospitalized mental patients, *Science*, **204**, 966.

Freud, S. (1955). Beyond the pleasure principle (1920), in *The Standard Edition of the Psychological Works of Sigmund Freud* (Ed. J. Strachey), The Hogarth Press, London, pp. 7–64.

Funch, D. P., and Marshall, J. (1983). The role of stress, social support and age in survival from breast cancer, *J. Psychosom. Res.*, **27**, 77.

Goldfarb, C., Driesen, J., and Cole, D. (1967). Psychophysiologic aspects of malignancy, *Am. J. Psychiat.*, **123**, 1545.

Greer, S., and Morris, T. (1975). Psychological attributes of women who develop breast cancer: A controlled study, *J. Psychosom. Res.*, **19**, 147.

Greer, S., and Morris, T. (1978). The study of psychological factors in breast cancer: Problems of method, *Soc. Sci. Med.*, **12**, 129.

Greer, S., Morris, T., and Pettingale, K. W. (1979). Psychological response to breast cancer: Effect on outcome, *Lancet*, **2**, 785.

Grinker, R. R. (1966). Psychosomatic aspects of the cancer problem, *Ann. NY Acad. Sci.*, **125**, 876.

Hagnell, O. (1966). The premorbid personality of persons who develop cancer in a total population investigated in 1947 and 1957, *Ann. NY Acad. Sci.*, **125**, 846.

Harris, J. R., Hellman, S., Cnellos, G. P., and Fisher, B. (1985). Cancer of the breast, in *Cancer—Principles & Practice of Oncology* (Eds V. T. DeVita, S. Hellman and S. Rosenberg), J. B. Lippincott, New York, pp. 1119–1177.

Harrison, R. F., O'Moore, R. R., and O'Moore, A. M. (1986). Stress and fertility: Some modalities of investigation and treatment in couples with unexplained infertility in Dublin, *Int. J. Fert.*, **31**, 153.

Helsing, K. J., Comstock, G. W., and Szklo, M. (1982). Causes of death in a widowed population, *Am. J. Epidem.*, **116**, 524.

Helsing, K. J., and Szklo, M. (1981). Mortality after bereavement, *Am. J. Epidem.*, **114**, 41.

Henderson, I. C., and Canellos, G. P. (1980a). Cancer of the breast, *New Eng. J. Med.*, **302**, 17.

Henderson, I. C., and Canellos, G. P. (1980b). Cancer of the breast, *New Eng. J. Med.*, **302**, 78.

Houck, J. C., and Attallah, A. M. (1975). Chalones (specific and endogenous mitotic inhibitors) and cancer, in *Cancer: A Comprehensive Treatise*, Vol. 3 (Ed. F. F. Becker), Plenum Press, New York, pp. 287–326.

Inman, W. S. (1967). Emotion, cancer and time: coincidence or determinism? *Brit. J. Med. Psych.*, **40**, 225.

Jansen, M. A., and Muenz, L. R. (1984). A retrospective study of personality variables associated with fibrocystic disease and breast cancer, *J. Psychosom. Res.*, **28**, 35.

Jones, D. R., Goldblatt, P. O., and Leon, D. A. (1984). Bereavement and cancer: some data on deaths of spouses from the longitudinal study of Office of Population Censuses and Surveys, *Brit. Med. J.*, **289**, 461.

Katz, J., Gallagher, T., Hellma, L., Sachar, E., and Weiner, H. (1969). Psychoendocrine considerations in cancer of the breast, *Ann. NY Acad. Sci.*, **164**, 509.

Katz, J. L., Ackman, P., Rothwax, Y., Sachar, E. J., Weiner, H., Hellman, L., and Gallagher, T. F. (1970). Psychoendocrine aspects of cancer of the breast, *Psychosom. Med.*, **32**, 1.

Kavetsky, R. E., Turkevich, N. M., and Balitsky, K. P. (1966). On the psychophysiological mechanism of the organism's resistance to tumor growth, *Ann. NY Acad. Sci.*, **125**, 933.

Ketcham, A. S., and Sindelar, W. F. (1975). Risk factors in breast cancer, in *Progress in Clinical Cancer* (Ed. I. M. Ariel), Grune & Stratton, New York, pp. 99–114.

Klopfer, B. (1957). Psychological variables in human cancer, *J. Proj. Tech.*, **21**, 331.

Kowal, S. J. (1955). Emotions as a cause of cancer, *Psychoanal. Rev.*, **42**, 217.

Krasnoff, A. (1959). Psychological variables and human cancer: A cross-validation study, *Psychosom. Med.*, **21**, 291.

Krippner, S., and Rubin, D. (Eds) (1973). *Galaxies Of Life: The Human Aura in Acupuncture and Kirlian Photography*, Gordon and Breach, New York.

Kushner, H. S. (1981). *When Bad Things Happen to Good People*, Avon Books, New York.

LeShan, L. (1959). Psychological states as factors in the development of malignant disease. *J. Nat. Cancer Inst.*, **22**, 1.

LeShan, L. (1960). Some methodological problems in the study of the psychosomatic aspects of cancer, *J. Gen. Psychol.*, **63**, 309.

LeShan, L. (1961). A basic psychological orientation apparently associated with malignant disease, *Psych. Quart.*, **35**, 314.

LeShan, L. (1966). An emotional life-history pattern associated with neoplastic disease, *Ann. NY Acad. Sci.*, **125**, 780.

LeShan, L. (1977). *You Can Fight For Your Life*, M. Evans & Company, New York.

LeShan, L., and Reznikoff, M. (1960). A psychological factor apparently associated with neoplastic disease, *J. Abn. Soc. Psych.*, **60**, 439.

LeShan, L., and Worthington, R. E. (1955). Some psychologic correlates of neoplastic disease: A preliminary report, *J. Clin. Exp. Psychopath.*, **16**, 281.

LeShan, L., and Worthington, R. E. (1956a). Personality as a factor in the pathogenesis of cancer: A review of the literature, *Brit. J. Med. Psych.*, **29**, 49.

LeShan, L., and Worthington, R. E. (1956b). Some recurrent life history patterns observed in patients with malignant disease, *J. Nerv. Ment. Dis.*, **124**, 460.

LeShan, L., and Worthington, R. E. (1956c). Loss of cathexes as a common psychodynamic characteristic of cancer patients: An attempt at statistical validation of a clinical hypothesis, *Psychol. Rep.*, **2**, 183.

Levy, S. M. (1985). *Behavior and Cancer: Life-Style and Psychosocial Factors in the Initiation and Progression of Cancer*, Jossey-Bass, San Francisco.

Levy, S. M., Herberman, R. B., Maluish, A. M., Schlien, B., and Lippman, M. (1985). Prognostic risk assessment in primary breast cancer by behavioral and immunological parameters, *Health Psychol.*, **4**, 99.

Lobo, R. A., Granger, L. R., Paul, W. L., Goebelsmann, U., and Mishell, D. R. (1983). Psychological stress and increases in urinary norepinephrine metabolites, platelet serotonin, and adrenal androgens in women with polycystic ovary syndrome, *Am. J. Obstet. Gynecol.*, **145**, 496.

Locke, S. E., Kraus, L., Leserman, J., Hurst, M. W., Heisel, S., and Williams, R. M. (1984). Life change stress, psychiatric symptoms, and natural killer cell activity, *Psychosom. Med.*, **46**, 441.

Maguire, P. (1979). The will to live in the cancer patient, in *Mind and Cancer Prognosis* (Ed. B. A. Stoll), John Wiley & Sons, New York, pp. 169–182.

Mason, J. W. (1975). Psychologic stress and endocrine function, in *Topics In Psychoendocrinology* (Ed. E. J. Sachar), Grune & Stratton, New York, pp. 1–18.

Miller, A. B., and Bulbrook, R. D. (1980). The epidemiology and etiology of breast cancer, *New Eng. J. Med.*, **303**, 1246.

Moeller, G., and Moeller, E. (1975). Considerations of some current concepts in cancer research, *J. Nat. Cancer Inst.*, **55**, 755.

Moore, D. H., Moore, D. H., and Moore, C. T. (1983). Breast carcinoma etiological factors, *Adv. Cancer Res.*, **40**, 189.

Morris, T., Greer, S., Pettingale, K. W., and Watson, M. (1981). Patterns of expression of anger and their psychological correlates in women with breast cancer, *J. Psychosom. Res.*, **25**, 11.

Muslin, H. L., Gyarfas, K., and Pieper, W. J. (1966). Separation experience and cancer of the breast, *Ann. NY Acad. Sci.*, **125**, 802.

Nagington, J., and Rook, A. (1979). Virus and related infections, in *Textbook of Dermatology* (Eds A. Rook and D. S. Wilkinson), Blackwell Scientific Publications, Oxford, pp. 607–676.

Ostrander, S., and Schroeder, L. (1970). *Psychic Discoveries Behind the Iron Curtain*, Prentice-Hall, Englewood Cliffs.

Overall, J. E. (1978). Prior psychiatric treatment and the development of breast cancer, *Arch. Gen. Psych.*, **35**, 898.

Paget, J. (1871). *Lectures On Surgical Pathology*, Lindsay & Blakiston, Philadelphia.

Pardee, A. B. (1985). Principles of cancer biology: Biochemistry and cell biology, in *Cancer—Principles & Practice of Oncology* (Eds V. T. DeVita, S. Hellman and S. Rosenberg), J. B. Lippincott, New York, pp. 3–22.

Parker, L., Eugene, E., Farber, D., Lifrak, E., Lai, M., and Juler, G. (1985). Dissociation of adrenal androgen and cortisol levels in actue stress, *Horm. Metab. Res.*, **17**, 209.

Pass, F. (1982). Warts: Virology, immunology, and therapy, in *Dermatology Update* (Ed. S. L. Moschella), Elsevier, New York, pp. 1–13.

Perrin, G. M., and Pierce, I. R. (1959). Psychosomatic aspects of cancer, *Psychosom. Med.*, **21**, 397.

Peters, L. J., and Mason, K. A. (1979). Influence of stress on experimental cancer, in *Mind and Cancer Prognosis* (Ed. B. A. Stoll), John Wiley & Sons, New York, pp. 103–124.

Pettingale, K. W., Greer, S., Morris, T., and Haybittle, J. L. (1985). Mental attitudes to cancer: An additional prognostic factor, *Lancet*, **1**, 750.

Pettingale, K. W., Greer, S., and Tee, D. E. H. (1977). Serum IgA and emotional expression in breast cancer patients, *J. Psychosom. Res.*, **21**, 395.

Pitot, H. C. (1985). Principles of cancer biology: Chemical carcinogenesis, in *Cancer—Principles & Practice of Oncology* (Eds V. T. DeVita, S. Hellman and S. Rosenberg), J. B. Lippincott, New York, pp. 79–99.

Priestman, T. J., Priestman, S. G., and Bradshaw, C. (1985). Stress and breast cancer, *Brit. J. Cancer*, **51**, 493.

Rakoff, A. E. (1962). Psychogenic factors in anovulatory women, *Fert. Ster.*, **13**, 1.

Rather, L. J. (1978). *The Genesis Of Cancer—A Study in the History of Ideas*, Johns Hopkins University Press, Baltimore.

Renneker, R. E., Cutler, R., Hora, J., Bacon, C., Bradley, G., Kearney, J., and Cutler, M. (1963). Psychoanalytical explorations of emotional correlates of cancer of the breast, *Psychosom. Med.*, **25**, 106.

Reznikoff, M. (1955). Psychological factors in breast cancer, *Psychosom. Med.*, **17**, 96.

Reznikoff, M., and Martin, D. E. (1957). The influence of stress on mammary cancer in mice, *J. Psychosom. Res.*, **2**, 56.

Riffenburgh, R. H. (1969). A speculative mathematical model of the psychophysiologic system, *Ann. NY Acad. Sci.*, **164**, 409.

Rose, R. M., Bourne, P. G., Poe, R. O., Mougey, E. H., Collins, D. R., and Mason, J. W. (1969). Androgen response to stress—II, *Psychosom. Med.*, **31**, 418.

Scheflen, A. E. (1951). Malignant tumors in the institutionalized psychotic population, *Arch. Neur. Psych.*, **66**, 145.

Schonfield, J. (1975). Psychological and life-experience differences between Israeli women with benign and cancerous breast lesions, *J. Psychosom. Res.*, **19**, 229.

Seligson, T. (1987). 'We don't lie to each other', *Parade Magazine*, 11 January, 8.

Shekelle, R. B., Raynor, W. J., Ostfeld, A. M., Garron, D. C., Bieliauskas, L. A., Liu, S. C., Maliza, C., and Paul, O. (1981). Psychological depression and 17-year risk of death from cancer, *Psychosom. Med.*, **43**, 117.

Shrifte, M. L. (1962). Toward identification of a psychological variable in host resistance to cancer, *Psychosom. Med.*, **24**, 390.

Siegel, R. E. (1968). *Galen's System of Physiology and Medicine*, S. Karger, New York.

Simonton, O. C., and Matthews-Simonton, S. (1981). Cancer and stress: Counselling the cancer patient, *Med. J. Aust.*, **1**, 679.

Simonton, O. C., Matthews-Simonton, S., and Creighton, J. (1978). *Getting Well Again*, J. P. Tarcher, Los Angeles.

Sinclair-Gieben, A. H. C. (1959). Evaluation of treatment of warts by hypnosis, *Lancet*, **2**, 480.

Sklar, L. S., and Anisman, H. (1979). Stress and coping factors influence tumor growth, *Science*, **205**, 513.

Sklar, L. S., and Anisman, H. (1981). Stress and cancer, *Psychol. Bull.*, **89**, 369.

Smith, W. R., and Sebastian, H. (1976). Emotional history and pathogenesis of cancer, *J. Clin. Psychol.*, **32**, 863.

Snell, L., and Graham, S. (1971). Social trauma as related to cancer of the breast, *Brit. J. Cancer*, **25**, 721.

Stavraky, K. M. (1968). Psychological factors in the outcome of human cancer, *J. Psychosom. Res.*, **12**, 251.

Stefansson, V. (1960). *Cancer: Disease of Civilization*, Hill & Wang, New York.

Stoll, B. A. (1979a). Is Hope a Factor in Survival?, in *Mind and Cancer Prognosis* (Ed. B. A. Stoll), John Wiley & Sons, New York, pp. 183–197.

Stoll, B. A. (1979b). Restraint of growth and spontaneous regression of cancer, in *Mind and Cancer Prognosis* (Ed. B. A. Stoll), John Wiley & Sons, New York, pp. 19–29.

Stoll, B. A. (1985). Psychoendocrine pathways and cancer prognosis, in *Psychological Aspects of Cancer* (Ed. M. Watson *et al.*), Pergamon Press, Oxford.

Stutman, O. (1983). The immunological surveillance hypothesis, in *Basic and Clinical Tumor Immunology* (Ed. R. B. Herberman), Martinus Nijhoff, Boston, pp. 1–81.

Tarlau, M., and Smalheiser, I. (1951). Personality patterns in patients with malignant tumors of the breast and cervix, *Psychosom. Med.*, **13**, 117.

Thomas, C. B. (1976). Precursors of premature disease and death, *Ann. Int. Med.*, **85**, 653.

Thomas, C. B., and Duszynski, K. R. (1974). Closeness to parents and the family constellation in a prospective study of five disease states: Suicide, mental illness, malignant tumor, hypertension and coronary heart disease, *Hopkins Med. J.*, **134**, 251.

Thomas, C. B., Duszynski, K. R., and Shaffer, J. W. (1979). Family attitudes reported in youth as potential predictors of cancer, *Psychosom. Med.*, **41**, 287.

Thomas, C. B., and Greenstreet, R. L. (1973). Psychobiological characteristics in youth as predictors of five disease states: Suicide, mental illness, hypertension, coronary heart disease and tumor, *Hopkins Med. J.*, **132**, 16.

Ultmann, J. E., and Golomb, H. M. (1983). Principles of neoplasia: Approach to diagnosis and management, in *Harrison's Principles of Internal Medicine*, 10th edn (Ed. R. G. Petersdorf), McGraw-Hill, New York, pp. 751–764.

Viitamaki, R. O. (1970). Psychological determinants of cancer, in *Cancer And Psyche*, Monographs from the Psychiatric Clinic of Helsinki, **1**, 45–142.

Voth, H. M. (1976). Cancer and personality, *Percept. Mot. Skills*, **42**, 1131.

Walshe, W. H. (1846). *The Nature and Treatment of Cancer*, Taylor & Walton, London.

Watson, C. G., and Schuld, D. (1977). Psychosomatic factors in the etiology of neoplasms, *J. Consulting Clin. Psychol.*, **45**, 455.

Weisman, A. D., and Worden, J. W. (1975). Psychosocial analysis of cancer deaths, *Omega*, **6**, 61.

West, P. M., Blumberg, E. M., and Ellis, F. W. (1952) An observed correlation between psychological factors and growth rate of cancer in man, *Cancer Res.*, **12**, 306.

Wheeler, J. I., and Caldwell, B. M. (1955). Psychological evaluation of women with cancer of the breast and of the cervix, *Psychosom. Med.*, **17**, 256.

Section Three
Psychosocial Factors and the Progression of Breast Cancer

Stress and Breast Cancer
Edited by C. L. Cooper
© 1988 John Wiley & Sons Ltd

Chapter 3
Breast Cancer: Psychological Factors Influencing Progression

Maggie Watson
Senior Research Psychologist and Lecturer, CRC Psychological Medicine Research Group, The Royal Marsden Hospital and Institute of Cancer Research, Surrey, UK

PSYCHOLOGICAL FACTORS IN BREAST CANCER PROGRESSION

A great deal has been written about the possible role of stress in the onset and progression of cancer. The topic is certainly not new and some of the earliest references to psychological characteristics of women developing cancer were attributed to Galen, a physician during the second century (Mettler and Mettler, 1947). Examining the relationship between stress and cancer has remained notoriously difficult because of the complexity of the biological processes and our limited understanding of carcinogenesis. Despite this, psychobiological models have been proposed, with immunosuppression currently being favoured as a possible process linking stress with cancer. The model we have followed for the last decade (Pettingale, 1985; Greer and Watson, 1985) was influenced by the theory of immunosurveillance proposed by Burnet (1957) (Figure 1). Little was known about the interaction between 'stress hormones' and immune function a decade or so ago but they have subsequently been shown to be interlinked (Besedovsky and Sorkin, 1981), thereby providing a feasible biological basis on which to work. Looking more closely at this model, 'psychological factors' has been taken to mean those components of individuals' behaviour which somehow act to mediate their responses to stressful events (i.e. stressors). Within the literature these psychological factors have been described variously as personality dimensions, coping responses or attitudes. Nevertheless, there is generally considered to be something about the psychological responses of some individuals which makes them feel particularly vulnerable to distress. Such 'stress-prone' individuals will have more circulating stress hormones and these

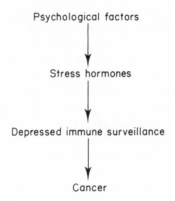

Figure 1: A psychoimmunological
model of breast cancer.

interact with immunological responses to depress the competence of the immune system. This depression in immune competence or surveillance prevents components of the body's defence system from functioning to inhibit either carcinogenesis or cancer cell reproduction.

The idea that stress or psychological responses might be linked to breast cancer is not new but until recently has not received any serious consideration and, indeed, is still considered by 'hard-nosed' oncologists to be of little importance. However, the last decade of research in psychoneuro-immunology has at least allowed a possible model which might explain the stress–cancer link. Some caution is needed, however, as a number of problems exist in the model described. For instance, the evidence for a cancer-prone personality type remains extremely flimsy. A review by Fox (1976) indicated that the findings remain contradictory. There certainly seem to be differences between the psychological responses of breast cancer patients and controls (Morris *et al.*, 1981; Watson, Pettingale and Greer, 1984) but it is not easy, in the absence of large scale prospective studies, to say how important these might be in the process of carcinogenesis. The timing of studies measuring psychological factors may also be crucial. Brain and Henson (1958) have indicated that disturbances of mood and neurological abnormalities could antedate the *appearance* of carcinoma by at least three years. This view was confirmed in a study by Kerr and colleagues (Kerr, Schapira and Roth, 1969) in which depressive illness, developing in men of late middle age without previous psychiatric illness, was subsequently found to be a possible early indication of malignant disease. There are clearly methodological problems in this area which prevent any firm conclusions about the role of psychological responses in carcinogenesis.

Following the model through, we have the idea that stress may be immunosuppressive. Yet, there are numerous possible biological mechanisms which can mediate the effects of stress on the malignant process. Pettingale (1985) has argued that the precise role of the immune system in tumour biology is still unclear. Recent findings on the role of oncogenes (Waterfield *et al.*, 1983) in carcinogenesis have caused a revision in the role of the immune system in the earliest transformations of cells to a malignant state. It now seems unlikely the immune system could recognize such small quantitative changes in cells or that immune surveillance is involved in the detection of the earliest malignant changes. Although these early changes may not be influenced by immunological processes, the growth of tumours and their metastatic spread might well be affected by the body's defence system. During the last decade there has been a substantial output of findings contributing to our knowledge of the immune system. These findings have emphasized its complexity but have also clearly indicated that the immunological and neuroendocrine systems are intimately linked, thereby providing the biological basis for a psychoneuro-immunological model of cancer progression. There would seem, therefore, to be strong arguments in favour of examining the possible role of psychological factors in cancer *progression*. At this point it might be useful to review the evidence relating to psychological factors in cancer progression, in order to say if any discernible trends are emerging about the psychological attributes contributing to cancer prognosis.

To date only a limited number of studies have examined the possible links between psychological responses and cancer progression. So few studies exist relating to breast cancer that it is not possible to review trends for this group. Taking studies of all the different cancer types, these can be divided into two groups: those which relate to early stage disease and those which look at patients whose disease is widespread. In the former a number of studies deal with the link between psychological response and either incidence of metastases or rate of survival, whereas the latter have only survival as the main outcome criterion.

PSYCHOLOGICAL FACTORS IN EARLY STAGE DISEASE

One of the earliest studies (Katz *et al.*, 1970) examined hormone secretion in a group of women awaiting breast biopsy with the aim of determining whether shifts in psychological state correlated with stress hormone secretion ratios. They found that patients with relatively elevated hydrocortisone production rates displayed a variety of unpleasant affects. Those with relatively low rates showed responses such as hope, pride or humour. The low producers most frequently employed defences such as denial and rationalization and showed more faith in God, stoicism and fatalism. However, it was not possible to say if any one set of defences was invariably correlated with a specific range of hydrocortisone production. They drew attention to their observation that several of the breast cancer patients utilized the defence of denial. When such denial was effective, values for the production rate of hydrocortisone were low and ratios were more apt to fall into the 'good prognosis' category. Their results suggested that rate of stress hormone production might be affected by extreme psychological responses. No follow-up was reported in this study so it was not possible to see how such responses might relate to disease progression. To have a significant effect on disease status this would presumably need to be a chronic response. As yet no evidence exists relating to the long-term effects of these psychological responses on stress hormone production and subsequent disease progression.

Weisman and Worden (1977) studied five different groups of cancer patients: breast, colon, lung, Hodgkin's disease and melanoma. Eighty-two per cent of these had no evidence of metastases at the time of assessment. In order to study the effects of psychological response on survival, a survival quotient was calculated. Expected survival figures for each cancer site and stage were calculated from a large sample of patients. How the patients' observed survival deviated from the expected survival became the survival quotient. Patients were assessed within ten days of their first admission for treatment and where possible were followed up for a period of 18 months. Their sample was divided into either short or long survivors on the basis of the survival quotient and then compared on a number of psychological dimensions. Short survivors expressed more suicidal ideas, showed poorer resolution of problems, had higher peaks of vulnerability and expressed greater dissatisfaction with their medical progress. They were also more likely to fail to comply with medical directives and were considered 'uncooperative' patients. It would be interesting to know to what extent this latter tendency might have influenced their progress, that is, was failure to comply with treatment a factor influencing disease progression in this sample? Compared to this group, those showing a longer survival in relation to the survival quotient had lower peaks of vulnerability and showed a more positive response on all of the dimensions described above.

In a prospective study of women with early breast cancer (Greer, Morris and Pettingale, 1979) results indicated that psychological response assessed three months post-operatively was related to outcome five years later. Recurrence-free survival was significantly more common among patients who reacted to cancer by 'fighting spirit' or 'denial' than among patients who had responded with 'stoic acceptance' or 'helplessness/hopelessness'. A ten-year follow-up on the same group of patients indicated that a 'fighting spirit' was still significantly associated with a better prognosis (Pettingale *et al.*, 1985). These responses were assessed using a clinical interview at three months post-operatively with patients being allocated to a single category of response. No findings are yet available on the consistency of such responses but further research is in progress by this group, using standardized questionnaire techniques, which may clarify the consistency issue (Greer and Watson, 1987). These psychological responses were found to be independent of clinical prognostic indicators. The explanation for why an association exists between those attitudes to a cancer diagnosis and the rate of survival remains unclear but these findings suggest that such attitudes might be *additional* prognostic indicators in breast cancer. There is a need, however, to examine these responses using more manageable techniques than the clinical interview, with a view perhaps to measuring consistency or chronicity.

A study by Rogentine *et al*. (1979) identified a psychological variable which predicted the rate of one-year disease-free survival in a group of patients with Stage I and II malignant melanoma. This finding, like that of Greer and his colleagues, did not appear to be confounded by an association with any known biological prognostic factors. It was independent of the only such variable which did predict outcome, that is, the number of positive lymph nodes. The psychological response was measured on a single dimension, with patients being asked to rate the amount of personal adjustment needed to handle or cope with the surgery for melanoma. This was defined as the 'melanoma adjustment score'. Where a lot of adjustment was reported, the relapse rate was *lower*. They interpreted these data as indicating that those with a higher relapse rate had reduced emotional reactivity. However, the meaning of this single dimension measure is not clear. Also, when follow-up was extended to three years in this group, the melanoma adjustment score was no longer related to disease outcome (Temoshok and Fox, 1984). They made the point that if the illness has progressed too far psychological factors may not be related to survival. As with many other studies in this area, their data did not answer the question of whether the relationship between psychological characteristics and cancer was causal.

More recently one study (Di Clemente and Temoshok, 1985) partially replicated the Greer findings in a group with malignant melanoma. Most were early stage patients assessed within one month of biopsy and followed up for a period of 26 months. Two factors predicted increased risk of disease recurrence: tumour thickness and feelings of helplessness/hopelessness. An analysis for the sexes separately indicated that the responses of stoicism among women and helplessness/hopelessness among men were more likely to be related to higher relapse rates. However, the major prognostic determinant remained the biology of the tumour, especially tumour thickness. Using a matched design study, Temoshok *et al*. (1987) hypothesized that when patients were matched initially on important biological and demographic prognostic factors, those in the poor outcome group would be significantly different from those in the good outcome group. Using this slightly different approach, complete data were obtained on the psychological responses of thirteen patients who had metastases at follow-up and twelve with no evidence of disease. The striking finding was that unfavourable outcome was linked with significantly higher levels of negative mood around the time of biopsy. On all negative affect dimensions measured within one month of biopsy, the unfavourable outcome group was significantly or nearly significantly higher than patients with a favourable outcome. Given that the patients were initially matched on a number of important biological variables, including tumour thickness, these findings lend strong support to feelings of distress as influencing the course of this disease. The number of patients was very small, however, and such results need replicating with a larger sample.

PSYCHOLOGICAL FACTORS IN LATE STAGE DISEASE

Davies *et al.* (1973), studying patients with advanced disease, found that an attitude of 'apathetic–given up' correlated with shorter survival. Such patients showed greater dysphoric feelings of anxiety, depression and hostility. Shorter survival was also associated with a greater degree of illness and presence of a haematologic disorder. These results suggest that physical changes associated with advanced illness may strongly influence adjustment. The relationship between the psychological reaction and shorter survival is by no means simple and according to these authors the psychological state is a product of the disease process. Achterberg and Lawlis (1977) simply looked at whether any psychological variables were predictive of present disease status and status after a two-month follow-up. They examined a broad range of cancer types, classified overall as widely metastatic or incurable. The results indicated that patients with a poorer prognosis at the two months' follow-up (i.e. those with evidence of significant tumour growth) were more likely to show denial, perceive themselves as having little ability to fight the disease, and expressed a significant level of dependency on others.

It could be argued that such a short follow-up is of limited use when examining the influence of psychological responses upon the disease course. Even in studies with a longer follow-up there are difficulties in interpreting the data. Derogatis, Abeloff and Melisaratos (1979) examined outcome over a much longer period in a group of 35 women with metastatic breast cancer. Patients were designated short-term survivors if they died within one year of the baseline psychological assessment. Those surviving beyond one year were designated long-term survovors. A number of significant differences were observed in the psychological profiles of the two groups. Long-term survivors reported more feelings of hostility, psychoticism, depression and guilt. Overall, they appeared less well adjusted and held more negative attitudes towards their illness and its treatment. They did, however, report increased feelings of vigour relative to short-term survivors. Compared to these responses the short-term survivors had higher scores for joy, contentment and affection. The authors concluded that patients who died more rapidly appeared distinctly *less* able to communicate dysphoric feelings, particularly those of anger and hostility. They considered that 'cancer patients whose coping styles facilitate external, conscious expression of negative emotions and psychological distress, appear to survive longer'. These results should be interpreted with some caution. For instance, the authors highlight the inability of short-term survivors to express negative emotions. Yet on at least one dimension of negative affect reported, phobic anxiety, the short-term survivors did show a greater response, although not significantly so. The small numbers in this study also indicate some caution is needed in interpreting the results. More important, however, the two groups (i.e. long vs short survivors) had different degrees of treatment by chemotherapy. The short-term survivors had significantly *increased* exposure to chemotherapy, a mean of 407 days compared to 181 days for long-term survovors. This has two implications. It may have influenced length of survival and it may have influenced psychological response. Derogatis and colleagues argue that the increased exposure to chemotherapy in the short-term survivors might have suggested to these patients that progression of the cancer was imminent. The authors ask why it should be that these patients nevertheless show less dysphoric mood and are better adjusted to the illness. This is difficult to explain but there may be another interpretation of their results. It could be that the *decreased* exposure to chemotherapy in the long-term survivors was interpreted by them as an indication that the prognosis was poor (that is, 'I'm so ill the doctors have given up trying'). On a measure of the accuracy and quality of the patients' appreciation of their illness and its treatment, long-term survivors were found to be significantly *less* likely to have a positive attitude. Such a result might reflect the patients' perception that frequent aggressive treatment was not being undertaken *because* the prognosis was poor. Short-term survivors may have construed continuing treatment as an indication of hope. If this were correct, these differences in perception may account for the differences in the psychological profiles where short-term survivors showed less negative affect. Clearly the differences in treatment make it difficult to interpret their results and certainly the data cannot be taken as clear evidence that inhibition of negative emotions is related to shorter survival.

Finally, an important study by Cassileth *et al.* (1985) of patients with advanced disease found that psychological responses were unrelated to survival. The authors measured a wide range of variables which had been mentioned in the literature as being related to prognosis. Three hundred and fifty-nine patients were examined, including a subgroup of Stage II breast cancer patients. For the purposes of their analysis patients were divided into two groups: unresectable cancers—Group 1—and intermediate (e.g. Stage I and II melanoma and Stage II breast cancer)—Group 2. It was not clear why early stage breast cancer patients were excluded from their study but presumably it was because of the long follow-up required for these patients. Group 1 was examined in terms of relationship of psychosocial factors to length of survival, whereas patients in Group 2 were followed to time of recurrence of disease. Social and psychological factors did not influence either length of survival or time to relapse. Earlier stage patients were not studied and the authors state that they did not address the question of whether psychosocial factors might influence the outcome for patients with more favourable cancer diagnoses. They concluded that biological aspects of the disease predominate and override the potential influence of psychosocial variables once the disease process is well established.

There are a few studies where details of disease stage are either not included or have not been taken into account. One large study of breast cancer patients (Stavraky, 1968) found that the group with the most favourable outcome differed from others in that they had strong hostile drives but without any loss of emotional control. The patients with the most favourable outcome appeared to be the antithesis of those showing a giving-up reaction, with the expression of hostile responses relating to increased survival. It is becoming increasingly significant that disease stage is important in this area of research and their failure to take into account such an important variable obscures interpretation of these data. The study by Shrifte (1962) is also difficult to interpret because although patients were described as being 'ambulatory' at the time of assessment, disease stage is unclear.

There is one group of studies of particular interest. These are studies where psychological interventions have occurred, in the form of therapy/counselling, and the effects upon survival observed. Such experimental studies are interesting and would seem to have an increasingly important role in this research area. Most reports in this area can, however, be immediately discounted on the basis that no scientific evaluation was made of the effects of the psychological therapies. Frequently, case reports are given which provide anecdotal evidence supporting the authors' view. A few studies use larger numbers of patients. The work by Simonton, Matthews-Simonton and Sparks (1980) has attracted particular attention, especially from those interested in 'alternative medicine'. The authors have described the effects of their psychotherapy upon a large group of patients with advanced malignancy, including breast cancer. Patients were followed up for a minimum of two years and their length of survival compared to the median survival rates reported in a number of studies. They noted that their patients survived for a median period of 35 months compared to the average survival rate of sixteen months reported in the literature. There are a number of problems with this study. For instance, no assessment of psychological morbidity was made in order to determine whether their therapeutic intervention had any effect upon levels of depression or anxiety. Indeed, no statistical analyses are reported at all. There was no control group and no control was made for any effects due to the different medical treatments patients received.

Grossarth-Maticek (1980) also reported that one of the benefits of psychotherapy was increased survival. However, only a few patients were studied, no control was operated for stage or type of disease and length of follow-up was not clear. There is one outstanding study in this area (Linn, Linn and Harris, 1982) and their results indicated no benefit to patients in terms of increased survival as a result of counselling. Five cancer groups were selected (lung, colon, stomach, pancreas, prostate) all of which were clinical stage IV with an estimated survival of 3–12 months. They found that depression was significantly decreased as a result of counselling when this was assessed at the three-month follow-up but not at subsequent follow-ups. There were differences in reported quality of life as a result of therapy but this did not affect survival. They had hypothesized that if patients felt better as a result of the psychological therapy then survival might be extended. This did not occur. They concluded that 'if the disease process is far advanced intervention of any kind probably has relatively little impact on survival'. They go on to say that psychosocial intervention at an earlier stage might significantly influence survival. At present no study exists which satisfies scientific criteria *and* demonstrates that psychological therapies have any effect on either survival or rate of disease progression. Despite this, the experimental manipulation of psychological responses through appropriate psychological therapies represents an exciting challenge to those interested in examining the stress and breast cancer issue.

The question raised earlier was whether it was possible to discern any trends in the research findings linking psychological responses to prognosis. There are a few threads running through the work which provide some clues for future directions. For late stage cancer patients, that is those with metastases, there seems to be little supportive evidence for a link between certain psychological responses and increased length of survival. If there is any consensus it appears to be that, where the disease is firmly established, it is biological rather than psychological variables which influence length of survival. For patients whose disease is at an earlier stage there is some indication that psychological responses may represent an *additional* prognostic indicator. Increased distress, depression and feelings of helplessness and hopelessness have been linked with a poorer prognosis although direction of causality is still an open question. It may be, of course, that these responses do not *increase* the rate of disease progression but rather that positive, 'fighting' responses enhance or extend length of survival. This too remains unclear.

In many instances throughout the studies described here, it has been difficult to tease out whether it is *pathological* responses which may be important or more positive attitudes. It is often assumed that the presence of distress may be the key in the psychobiological model of stress and breast cancer. That, somehow, being stressed might reduce length of survival. Perhaps it is possible to be provocative here and suggest we might also consider whether positive, healthy responses increase length of survival. Often clinicians with a long experience of working with cancer patients can tell of some patients who, by usual clinical criteria, ought to be dead, but instead they have said 'Cancer isn't going to beat me', and have survived for longer than expected. The tantalizing question is how. As research in this area continues, hopefully this type of phenomenon will become explicable. For stress and breast cancer prognosis much research remains to be done. Further clarification is needed of the psychological responses and this issue needs to be pursued in parallel with research on the role of immunosurveillance and NK cell activity in breast cancer prognosis.

ACKNOWLEDGEMENTS

I would like to acknowledge Dr Steven Greer, Dr Keith Pettingale and Tina Morris, with whom I have worked over the last few years and with whom I have had many stimulating discussions about the issues outlined in this chapter.

REFERENCES

Achterberg, J., and Lawlis, G. F. (1977). Psychological factors and blood chemistries as disease outcome predictors for cancer patients, *Multivar. Exp. Clin. Res.*, **3**, 107–122.

Besedovsky, H. D., and Sorkin, E. (1981). *Psychoneuroimmunology* (Ed. R. Ader), Academic Press, New York, 545–574.

Brain, W. R., and Henson, R. A. (1958). Neurological syndromes associated with carcinoma, *Lancet*, **ii**, 971–975.

Burnet, F. M. (1957). Cancer—a biological approach, *Brit. Med. J.*, **1**, 779–786.

Cassileth, B. R., Lusk, E. J., Miller, D. S., Brown, L. L., and Miller, C. (1985). *New Eng. J. Med.*, **312**, 1551–1555.

Davies, R. K., Quinlan, D. M., McKegney, F. P., and Kimball, C. P. (1973). Organic factors and psychological adjustment in advanced cancer patients, *Psychosom. Med.*, **35**, 465–471.

Derogatis, L. R., Abeloff, M. D., and Melisaratos, N. (1979). Psychological coping mechanisms and survival time in metastatic breast cancer, *Am. Med. Assoc.*, **242**, 1504–1508.

Di Clemente, R. J., and Temoshok, L. (1985). Psychological adjustments to having cutaneous malignant melanoma as a predictor of follow up clinical status, *Psychosom. Med.*, **47**, 81.

Fox, B. H. (1976). The psychosocial epidemiology of cancer, in *Cancer: The Behavioural Dimension* (Eds J. W. Cullen, B. H. Fox and R. N. Isom), Raven Press, New York.

Greer, S., Morris, T., and Pettingale, K. W. (1979). Psychological response to breast cancer: effect on outcome, *Lancet*, **ii**, 785–787.

Greer, S., and Watson, M. (1985). Towards a psychobiological model of cancer: psychological considerations, *Soc. Sci. Med.*, **20**, 773–777.

Greer, S., and Watson, M. (1987). Mental adjustment to cancer: its management and prognostic importance, *Cancer Surv.*, in press.

Grossarth-Maticek, R. (1980). Social psychotherapy and course of the disease, *Psychother. Psychosomat.*, **33**, 129–138.

Katz, J. L., Ackerman, P., Rothwax, Y., Sachar, E. J., Weiner, H., Hellman, L., and Gallagher, T. F. (1970). Psychoendocrine aspects of cancer of the breast, *Psychosom. Med.*, **32**, 1–18.

Kerr, T. A., Schapira, K., and Roth, M. (1969). The relationship between premature death and affective disorders, *Brit. J. Psychiat.*, **115**, 1277–1282.

Linn, M. W., Linn, B. S., and Harris, R. (1982). Effects of counselling for late stage cancer patients, *Cancer*, **49**, 1048–1055.

Mettler, C. C., and Mettler, F. A. (1947). *History of Medicine*, Blakiston, Philadelphia.

Morris, T., Greer, S., Pettingale, K. W., and Watson, M. (1981). Patterns of expression of anger and their psychological correlates in women with breast cancer, *J. Psychosom. Res.*, **25**, 111–117.

Pettingale, K. W. (1985). A review of psychobiological interactions in cancer patients, in *Advances in the Biosciences Vol. 49. Psychological Aspects of Cancer* (Eds M. Watson and T. Morris), Pergamon Press, Oxford.

Pettingale, K. W., Morris, T., Greer, S., and Haybittle, J. L. (1985). Mental attitudes to cancer: an additional prognostic factor, *Lancet*, **i**, 750.

Rogentine, G. N., Van Kammen, D. P., Fox, B. H., Docherty, J. P., Rosenblatt, J. E., Boyd, S. C., and Bunney, W. E. (1979). Psychological factors in the prognosis of malignant melanoma: a prospective study, *Psychosom. Med.*, **41**, 647–655.

Shrifte, M. L. (1962). Toward identification of a psychological variable in host resistance to cancer, *Psychosom. Med.*, **24**, 390–397.

Simonton, O. C., Matthews-Simonton, S., and Sparks, T. F. (1980). Psychological intervention in the treatment of cancer, *Psychosomatics*, **21**, 226–233.

Stavraky, K. M. (1968). Psychological factors in the outcome of human cancer, *J. Psychosom. Res.*, **12**, 251–259.

Temoshok, L., and Fox, B. H. (1984). Coping styles and other psychosocial factors related to medical status and to prognosis in patients with cutaneous malignant melanoma, in *Impact of Psychoendocrine Systems on Cancer and Immunity* (Eds B. H. Fox and B. H. Newberry), C. J. Hogrefe, Toronto.

Temoshok, L., Sweet, D. M., Blois, M. S., and Sagebiel, R. W. (1987). Psychosocial factors related to outcome in cutaneous malignant melanoma: a matched sampler design. Submitted to Journal of the American Medical Association.

Waterfield, M. D., Scrace, G. T., Whittle, N., Stroobant, P., Johnsson, A., Waterson, A., Westermark, B., Heldin, C-H., Huang, J. S., and Devel, T. F. (1983). Platelet-derived growth factor is structurally related to the putative transforming protein p28[sis] of simian sarcoma virus, *Nature*, **304**, 35–39.

Watson, M., Pettingale, K. W., and Greer, S. (1984). Emotional control and autonomic arousal in breast cancer patients, *J. Psychosom. Res.*, **28**, 467–474.

Weisman, A. D., and Worden, J. W. (1977). Coping and vulnerability in cancer patients. Privately printed, Boston, Mass.

Stress and Breast Cancer
Edited by C. L. Cooper
© 1988 John Wiley & Sons Ltd

Chapter 4
Psychosocial Risk Factors and Cancer Progression

Sandra M. Levy
and
Beverly D. Wise
Pittsburgh Cancer Institute, University of Pittsburgh School of Medicine, Pennsylvania, USA

The course of cancer varies. Given two individuals with biologically identical cancers, one might succumb to the disease rapidly while the other recovers with no further symptoms. How can this be explained? More importantly, what can we do to increase the number who recover? A large and varied literature supports the belief that psychosocial factors—an individual's feelings, thoughts, behaviors and social environment—play a significant role in disease course and outcome. Can we modify these variables and thereby have an impact on the course of an individual's cancer? Clinical trials and controlled, randomized experiments will eventually answer this question. As we shall demonstrate in this chapter, much of the preparatory work has been accomplished.

Anecdotal evidence that psychosocial factors are involved in the onset and course of cancer date back at least as far as early Greek writings. The story from the 1950s of a man with advanced lymphosarcoma is illustrative. The man was given an experimental drug called Krebiozen, for which both the man's physician and the lay press expressed high expectations. Amazingly, the man went into remission and resumed his normal activities. As the patient began to read reports of negative results with Krebiozen, however, he relapsed and became terminally ill. Hoping to reinvoke the patient's earlier response, the physician convinced the man that a new, purified form of Krebiozen *would* work. He injected a placebo, distilled water. And the patient again made a remarkable recovery. Only a few months later, the patient saw an authoritative governmental report declaring that Krebiozen was worthless. The man relapsed and died within a few weeks.

Other examples exist in which psychosocial events appear to have a negative impact on disease outcome. There are many cases in which a tumor is brought under control and has no impact on health for many years until a sudden trauma, such as a car accident or loss of a loved one, is followed by a recurrence of the tumor with dramatic deterioration of physical condition.

On the other hand, Stoll (1979) cites the case of a nun with pancreatic cancer for which the five-year survival rate is less than 1 per cent. The diagnosis was confirmed by three pathologists. Yet she grew stronger and went back to work after the other nuns in the order prayed for her. She died suddenly seven and a half years later. The autopsy revealed a massive embolism of the lung but no evidence of cancer.

In recent years the technology of both behavioral science and laboratory medicine have improved such that it has become possible to study systematically the relationships between behavior and cancer course. The first author launched a research program in this area in 1979 at the National Cancer Institute (NCI), National Institutes of Health, which continues today at the Pittsburgh Cancer Institute (PCI), University of Pittsburgh. Interdisciplinary collaborations have allowed us to explore not only relationships between psychosocial factors and disease outcomes, but also the biological mechanisms that appear most likely to mediate two-way communication between central nervous system pathways and peripheral cells and organs. Most of the work in this area has been focused on breast cancer and malignant melanoma.

This chapter will review the biological systems involved in this research and the evidence that central nervous system, endocrine and immune factors are associated with tumor course. We will then review findings from our research program of the last seven years. Finally, we will present a psychosocial model linking behavioral factors with cancer outcome.

CHOOSING TUMORS FOR STUDY

In attempting to understand the role of psychosocial variables in cancer course, it makes sense to study tumor systems in which such variables are most likely to be playing a substantial part, i.e. in cancers where biological factors may not account for total outcome variance. Both breast cancer and malignant melanoma have relatively unpredictable courses, at least in their intermediate stages. Very early and very advanced stages, as well as all stages of more virulent malignancies such as lung or pancreatic cancer, rarely deviate from their expected course. Thus, it is less likely the host's behavior will have a significant impact on disease course in the latter cases.

It also makes sense to study cancers for which there is a substantial range of response across individuals despite similar biological parameters and treatments. The variation then is most likely due to some unmeasured differences within individuals, possibly cortically mediated behavioral and social factors.

Again, breast cancer and malignant melanoma meet this criterion. Thus, these two tumor systems have been the most studied in this literature.

BREAST CANCER

Carcinoma of the breast is the most common malignancy in women, and it is slowly increasing in incidence and prevalence. It will strike approximately one out of every eleven females in the United States at some time in their lives. Despite gains in detection and treatment, the mortality rate has remained the same for the last half century (Keys, Bakermeier and Savlov, 1983).

MALIGNANT MELANOMA

Melanoma is a tumor originating in the melanocyte, a pigmented cell in the skin. Although still a relatively rare tumor, both incidence and mortality rates are rising rapidly in all countries where such records are kept. Mortality rates are rising by 3–9 per cent per year so that rates have doubled in the past fifteen years. Improved diagnosis and treatment have not greatly reduced these mortality rates. Treatment is by excision of the lesion; melanoma is virtually untreatable by radiation or chemotherapy at present (Carey, 1982). However, a disproportionate share of all cases of spontaneous regression have been reported for melanoma (e.g. Bodurtha *et al.*, 1976), suggesting endogenous host factors affecting tumor control. All these factors make it a good candidate for this research.

HORMONES AND CANCER

Although we will be concentrating on the relationships among malignancy, the brain and the immune system, it is important to remember that the neuroendocrine system is also part of the network that contributes to, and is affected by, changes in the other systems. Many studies have shown that hormone levels play an important part in contributing to breast cancer risk as well as the course of primary breast cancer and the growth of metastases (see, for example, Beatson, 1986; Lippman, 1985; Papatestas *et al.*, 1980).

The melanocyte—the cell from which melanomas derive—has a number of connecting pathways linking this cell with the endocrine system. It develops embryologically from the neural crest, and has a common origin with tissues that secrete peptide hormones or hormone-like substances such as gastrin, glucagon and ACTH. There have been reports of melanomas secreting serotonin. In addition, melanocyte-stimulating hormone arises from the same pituitary precursor molecule—proopiomelanocortin—as do ACTH and

B-endorphin, suggesting links among higher cortical function, hypothalamic pituitary hormone secretion and melanocyte activity.

IMMUNOLOGY

B cells, those lymphocytes which secrete antibodies in response to sensitization by a specific antigen, do not appear to play a large role in host defense against malignancy. Cytolytic T cells seem to be the major weapons in the body's fight with established tumors (Lewison, 1976; Pross and Baines, 1976; Cochran, 1978). And the macrophage serves in both a phagocytizing and a sensitizing capacity, in conjunction with T cells. However, tumor cells are very adaptive within an immunological environment (shedding antigens in the presence of antibodies against them, for example), and subpopulations of cells within heterogenous tumors have been reported to escape specific T-cell attack (Carey, 1982; Pross and Baines, 1976).

Natural killer (NK) cells are lymphocytes that have been shown to recognize and kill neoplastic cells without specific sensitization (Heberman and Santoni, 1984; Herberman and Holden, 1978). Such cells have been shown to kill heterogeneous tumor masses, including tumor emboli (Hanna and Fidler, 1980). Several *in vivo* models suggest that defects in NK activity can be correlated with increased susceptibility to malignancies, particularly lymphomas (Hanna and Fidler, 1980).

Other evidence for the importance of NK activity includes negative correlations between NK activity levels and growth of transplanted tumors in animal models (Hanna and Fidler, 1980; Herberman and Ortaldo, 1981). Likewise, susceptibility to spontaneous mammary tumors in C3H mice and spontaneous lymphomas in AKR mice correlate with low NK activity (Hanna, 1986). *In vitro*, NK cells have been shown to be cytolytic for a wide spectrum of malignant cells (leukemias, carcinomas, sarcomas and melanomas) (Sklar and Anisman, 1981; Lehman, Wortman and Williams, 1984).

IMMUNOLOGIC ASPECTS OF BREAST CANCER

Primary breast tumors have been reported to induce an immune response (Henderson and Cannellos, 1980; Humphrey, Singla and Volence, 1980). Studies looking at *in situ* and invasive breast carcinomas under the microscope have reported lymphoid cell infiltrations of the primary tumor (Nathanson, 1977; Moore and Foote, 1949). A recent study (Shimakowara *et al.*, 1982) showed that T-cell infiltration in breast tumors was scanty in scirrhous carcinoma but was ample in infiltrating papillotubular carcinoma, which has a better prognosis. There was also a significant inverse correlation between the intensity of the T-cell infiltration and clinical stage of disease, with advanced stage tumors showing practically no T-cell activity. And the intensity of the

T-cell infiltration was significantly higher in patients with no detectable lymph node metastases. Although these are only correlations, a causal connection is supported by animal experiments with autochthanous tumor systems (Kikochi *et al.*, 1976) that have demonstrated that some T-cell populations have a suppressive effect on cancer cell growth. In addition, we found a high correlation between depressed NK activity and spread of breast cancer to regional lymph nodes (Levy *et al.*, 1985).

IMMUNOLOGIC ASPECTS OF MELANOMA

Spontaneous regression of melanoma is sometimes associated with infection and may be characterized by the presence of lymphoid infiltrates within tumor tissue (Pross, 1986). This suggests that tumor cells are affected by general activation of the host's immune system.

The most common form of melanoma is the superficial spreading type, representing 60 per cent of all melanomas. It has a biphasic evolution, with a relatively slow horizontal growth phase followed by a rapid vertical penetration. Metastasis coincides with the vertical phase. There is commonly a dense lymphocyte infiltrate during the horizontal phase; a much weaker lymphocyte infiltration accompanies the vertical phase (Carey, 1982).

Recent *in vitro* studies with melanoma patients have shown decreased NK activity relative to normals that was also significantly correlated with more advanced stage of disease (Hersey, Edmond and McCarthy, 1980; Steinhauer *et al.*, 1982). Kadish *et al.* (1981) concluded that NK functional decrease seemed not to be secondary to suppressor cell activity. Response to interferon, normally an NK enhancer, was also impaired in patients with advanced disease. The number of effector-to-target conjugates was normal, even in patients with depressed NK function. However, the number of active lytic effectors was decreased. These results implied that the cells which bind tumor targets are present in patients with advanced melanoma, but these cells are either immature or functionally inactive.

Hersey, Edmond and McCarthy (in Reif and Mitchell, 1985) found differential changes in NK activity for melanoma patients with Stage I versus Stage II (more advanced) disease. For the Stage I patients, NK activity—which appeared to be directed specifically at melanoma cells—was maximal two to four weeks after removal of the tumor; it then decreased to normal levels. NK activity after surgery was positively correlated with thickness of the primary tumor. With the more advanced patients, in contrast, NK activity did not increase after surgery, but fell to low levels. There was no correlation between postsurgery NK activity and tumor thickness. The authors concluded that the differential NK activity following surgery in the two patient groups may have reflected differences in host response which contributed to spread of tumor to regional lymph nodes in the patients with poorer prognosis.

Recent work by Hanna and Colleagues (Hanna and Fidler, 1980; Hanna and Barton, 1981) has definitively demonstrated in an *in vivo* model that NK cells can inhibit tumor metastases, including circulating tumor emboli from a transplanted melanoma cell line. Therefore, the weight of recent clinical and experimental evidence suggests that NK cells play a significant role in controlling the spread of malignant melanoma.

Recent studies (Strayer, Carter and Brodsky, unpublished; Strayer *et al.*, 1984) of healthy women with a family history of breast cancer, and of individuals with high familial incidences of various cancers, including melanoma, showed significantly reduced NK cytotoxicity when compared to individuals without such a family history. Clinical studies (e.g. Lotzova and Herberman, 1986) indicate that patients with a variety of advanced cancers (including breast cancer and melanoma) had less NK activity against K562 target cells than those with localized malignancies. Of note, the number of NK cells (as determined by monoclonal antibody) was normal, but the functional killing capacity was reduced.

With advancing disease, however, there appears to be a decrease in immunological activity, due perhaps to lack of competent, sensitized cells, lack of tissue antigenicity, or both. One explanation for lack of containment of tumor cells is that those that 'slip through' are antigenically modified and thus escape detection and lysis by effector cells.

SYSTEM INTERACTIONS

Accumulating evidence indicates that the nervous system can exercise considerable control over the immune system (Del Rey, Besedovsky and Sorkin, 1984), and that proteins produced by monocytes modulate glucocorticoid blood levels and ACTH by way of the pituitary–adrenal axis (Besedovsky *et al.*, 1986). Among the possible mediators of cortical–immune interactions are neuropeptides and hormones (such as the steroids and catecholamines). Corticosteroids have been shown to modulate NK activity, perhaps due to a direct effect on NK cells or an indirect effect such as enhancement of suppressor cell activity. (For a good review, see the recent supplement to the *Journal of Immunology*, 1985.)

Lymphocytes have been shown to have receptors for a wide range of neuropeptides, including met-enkephalin. They also produce hormone-like substances (e.g. lymphokines such as interferon). Blalock (1984) has argued that the central nervous system and the immune system actually have non-cognitive sensory functions in the organism. They share common peptide signals (e.g. ACTH produced by both lymphocytes and the pituitary), common receptors (e.g. for the same neuropeptides) and common functions (e.g. lymphocyte products such as interferon can mimic hormone actions). Pert *et al.* (1985) have suggested that this 'psychoimmunoendocrine network'—cells in the brain, glands and immune system all communicating *via* the same chemicals and receptors—plays a major role in regulating vertebrate homeostasis.

THE NATIONAL CANCER INSTITUTE AND PITTSBURGH CANCER INSTITUTE PROGRAMS (1979–1986)

A report demonstrating an independent association between psychological factors and survival in advanced breast cancer patients (Derogatis, Abeloff and Melisaratos, 1979) prompted the first author to begin a systematic evaluation of the relationship. The series was started at the National Cancer Institute (NCI) and has continued at the Pittsburgh Cancer Institute (PCI). These studies, along with concurrent contributions from other researchers, have led us to formulate a model which will be presented later in this chapter.

1. Study of Survival in Advanced Breast Cancer Patients

A study of survival time in patients with advanced breast cancer (NCI Protocol 80-C-49) was initiated at the NCI (P.I., Dr Sandra Levy) in 1979. Thirty-four first-recurrent breast cancer patients (mean age = 52), having had no prior chemotherapy, participated in a structured interview, and reported mood symptoms using the Affect Balance Scale—a self-report of both positive and negative affect. Independent observers rated patients' psychological adjustment using the Global Adjustment to Illness Scale (GAIS) (Morrow, Chiarello and Derogatis, 1978), which has been shown to be a valid measure of psychological functioning in cancer patients (Morrow *et al.*, 1981). Interrater reliability on the GAIS was satisfactory ($r = 0.83$). Observers also rated patients on the Karnofsky Scale (Karnofsky and Burchenal, 1949), a standard measure of physical disability.

Biological indicators associated with length of survival were recorded from patients' charts. These included number and location of metastatic sites, number of local or regional lymph nodes positive for metastasis at time of diagnosis, disease-free interval (DFI) and age.

Baseline assessment was made shortly after the diagnosis of recurrence. Follow-up assessment occurred three months later, and patients have been followed since then until death. As of January 1987, 24 patients from the original sample have died, and we can now begin to answer the question originally posed: are psychological variables independently associated with survival time in this population?

When length of survival was split at one year beyond baseline, short survivors had significantly more nodes positive at original diagnosis ($t = 2.7$, $p < 0.01$), had delayed longer between detecting the original symptoms and seeking diagnosis ($t = 1.8$, $p < 0.08$), and had expressed less joy ($t = 1.9$,

$p < 0.07$) and more depression ($t = 1.7$, $p < 0.1$) at baseline assessment when compared with patients surviving a year or longer. When the split in length of survival was made at two years beyond baseline, long survivors had significantly more positive affect at baseline ($t = 2.3$, $p < 0.03$), had been rated at baseline by a physician as having a longer life expectancy ($t = 2.0$, $p < 0.05$), and had expressed significantly more joy ($t = 3.0$, $p < 0.009$) and less depression ($t = 1.8$, $p < 0.08$) than patients who died less than two years after our baseline assessment.

Using Cox's survival hazards model (Kalbfleisch and Prentise, 1980), DFI, number of metastatic sites, age and cell histology were entered into the stepwise analysis. We then entered psychological factors which were significantly associated with survival time (by t-test or Pearson correlations). A model combining DFI, joy, physician prognosis and number of metastatic sites proved to be the best predictor of survival time ($\chi^2 = 23.0$, $p < 0.0001$), with long DFI, more expressed joy, longer physician's prognosis and fewer metastatic sites associated with longer survival.

Joy is a surprising finding among women who have just learned that their breast cancer has recurred. This factor, which was derived from the ABS, probably shares a significant amount of variance with other biologically relevant variables, such as vigor and host resilience. Nevertheless, the psychosocial expression took the form of joy. Corroborating evidence comes from an epidemiological study carried out at the University of California at Berkeley (Reynolds and Kaplan, 1986). In the women of that cohort, wellbeing and happiness were predictive of a reduced incidence of cancer, and of decreased mortality, particularly from hormonally dependent tumors.

2. Study of Prognosis in Early Stage Breast Cancer Patients

We began collecting data on psychosocial factors and immune function of women undergoing treatment for primary disease at the NCI in 1981. As the initial findings have been published (Levy *et al.*, 1985), they will be summarized briefly here.

Subjects were interviewed and had blood taken after surgery but before the pathological findings were returned. It was found that NK activity in peripheral blood at this time predicted axillary lymph node status. Patients who had higher NK activity tended to have fewer lymph nodes with cancer. We then used a stepwise multiple regression analysis to look at the contribution of a number of psychosocial variables assessed concomitantly to NK activity variance. When the GAIS, the social support section of a structured interview, the Fatigue subscale of the Profile of Mood States (POMS) (McNair, Lorr and Droppleman, 1971), delay to diagnosis, total POMS score, age and overall SCL-90 index were entered into the equation, they accounted for 52 per cent of the variance in NK activity (F 3, 41 = 14.3, p

< 0.0001). However, the first three variables alone accounted for 51 per cent of the variance. Patients who were rated as well adjusted to their illness, who reported receiving less than desirable support from their environment and who expressed symptoms of fatigue tended to have lower NK activity levels. These findings have been replicated at three-month follow-up (Levy *et al.*, 1987).

3. Helplessness and Time to Recurrence in Early Stage Breast Cancer

We have been collaborating with Dr Martin Seligman (Department of Psychology, University of Pennsylvania) in an attempt to examine the effects of depressive pessimism and 'helplessness' in our sample of early breast cancer patients. Seligman and his colleagues have found that individuals who attribute negative events in their lives to internal, stable and global causes (that is, 'I caused it, this self-attribute is chronic in nature, and this "fatal flaw" will affect most aspects of my life') tend to be depressed and react with helplessness in the face of stressors (Spielberger *et al*, 1979). Seligman's Content Analysis of Verbatim Explanations (CAVE) (Peterson and Seligman, unpublished) allows us to go back to the interviews recorded with these patients and extract causal explanations that can then be analyzed according to a multidimensional helplessness construct. Does a helpless tendency predict recurrence of disease as the animal model of learned helplessness suggests?

Interview content of eight women with breast cancer recurrence was compared with that of eight non-recurrent controls, matched on time in treatment, treatment history and original nodal status. All causal explanations were rated blindly. We found that a number of helpless causal attributions were related to latency of recurrence. For example, internal attribution for negative social events happening to oneself showed a correlation of 0.71 with earlier recurrence ($p < 0.04$). In fact, almost all of the helplessness indices studied were associated in the expected direction with earlier disease recurrence.

We are continuing to follow the NCI samples, tabulating instances of recurrence and death. Final analyses will be performed in the next year. Meanwhile, the study has been expended at the University of Pittsburgh School of Medicine. We have added a measure of overnight urinary catecholamine excretion as a biological stress marker, and have expanded our battery of immunological tests. In addition, some refinements have been made in gathering psychosocial information. For example, we have expanded our assessment of social support to include the patients' perception of support from physicians, nurses and friends, as well as from family members. As of January 1987, we have 48 Stage I or II breast cancer patients active in this study. We expect to accrue a total of 120.

4. Pilot Study of Survival and Biological Vulnerability in Melanoma Patients and Healthy Normals

A pilot study of stress, coping and biological outcome in patients with advanced melanoma and normal volunteers (NCI Protocol 84-C-09) was initiated at the NCI as an outgrowth of the earlier breast cancer study. Here, too, we added the measurement of urinary catecholamine excretion to our biological assessment, and used the State–Trait Personality Inventory (STPI) (Spielberger *et al.*, 1979) as part of our psychosocial battery.

Despite a small sample of advanced melanoma patients ($N = 13$), we found very strong correlations between NK activity and distress indicators. Positive correlations were found between NK activity and trait curiosity ($+0.74$), vigor ($+0.70$), state anger ($+0.60$) and state curiosity ($+0.55$). Even more impressive negative correlations were found between NK activity and tension (-0.87), fatigue (-0.85), state anxiety (-0.69), total mood disturbance (-0.64) and depression (-0.61). One must be cautious when generalizing from such a small sample. However, these clusters of correlations are all in the expected direction, without a single anomaly among them. At the very least, the strengths of the associations are intriguing, and warrant further investigation.

Among the healthy volunteers, we identified a group at high risk for reporting more severe infectious illnesses at follow-up. It was found that these individuals had persistently low levels of NK activity at all three baseline measurements. They also tended to be younger than individuals with more normal NK variance, to report more 'hassles' in their daily lives and endorse fewer responses indicative of vigor. They had in addition significantly higher levels of norepinephrine (NE) excretion during baseline assessments. Similarly, Aoki's group (Aoki *et al.*, unpublished) has found increased incidence of illness among normal individuals who show reduced levels of NK activity over repeated testings. In fact, this Japanese group of investigators believe that they have discovered a new immunological disorder termed low NK syndrome. For Aoki and colleagues, the hallmark of this disease is complaints of fatigue and depressed mood. These findings support an expanded role for natural immunity in maintenance of a healthy state.

We are currently pursuing this line of investigation at the PCI. We will compare natural immunity profiles of normal, psychiatric and oncology populations, and develop behavioral and immunological intervention strategies aimed at enhancing immune function.

5. Enhancement of Functional Status in Colon Cancer and Melanoma Patients by a Cognitive Behavioral Intervention

We have just completed a pilot study, with collaborators at Yale University (Dr Judith Rodin) and at the University of Pennsylvania (Dr Martin

Seligman), examining the biological and psychological effects of a twelve-session therapeutic intervention designed to reduce depressogenic thought processes in cancer patients. Twenty-two patients with colon cancer and malignant melanoma were randomized to individual-treatment versus control conditions shortly after undergoing surgical excision of the primary lesion. Assessments were conducted at the beginning, middle and end of the twelve-week treatment time period. This project has primarily been a feasibility study, with the main purpose of refining our intervention for treatment of medical, non-psychiatric patients. In general, patients randomized to the treatment condition expressed more concerns over time, but became less helpless in terms of cognitive pessimism. Although the pilot sample was small, we are encouraged by these results and intend to launch a full-scale, prospective study, randomizing cancer patients to cognitive behavioral treatment versus a control condition, examining effects of treatment or immunological and disease parameters.

As we explore different populations with more sensitive assessment techniques, our research evolves. Ideas and hypotheses develop as we communicate not only with fellow members of a discipline, but with professionals and laypersons whose belief systems and technical vocabularies challenge some of our basic assumptions. When we succeed in joining these disparate elements together, old hypotheses are transformed and new ones are generated. Our successes to date have led us to investigate a particular coping style characterized as 'helpless', within a context of low familial support, which seems to characterize a biologically compromised population of cancer patients. NK activity has arisen as an important marker of host risk and has led us to discern, within a presumably normal population, a biologically vulnerable subgroup, characterized by persistently low NK activity values. As we pursue each of these leads, it is important to integrate the information obtained, always keeping in mind the question, 'So what?' A model helps us structure our observations.

PSYCHOSOCIAL RISK FACTORS: A MODEL

Table 1 provides a succinct overview of contemporary studies that have paved the way for our current and future research. The first two studies are epidemiological and concern the incidence of cancer; the other eight studies concern factors associated with progression or prognosis of established cancer. The third and fourth columns delineate the risk factors derived and the measures used to assess them.

It is apparent from Table 1 that few studies have measured the same constructs or used the same instruments, and a detailed review of this work is beyond the scope of this chapter. But three psychosocial factors associated with increased biological risk seem to emerge from the aggregate: inadequate

Table 1. Summary of Psychobiological Studies Linking Behavior and Cancer End-points

Investigator	Patients' and clinical end-point	Major constructs	Direction of association with worse outcome	Measures
1. Shekelle *et al.* 1981	All cancer mortality	Depression Other psychiatric variables	← →	MMPI
2. Reynolds and Kaplan 1986	All cancer incidence and mortality	Social isolation and unhappiness	←	Social Network Index
3. Derogatis *et al.* 1979	Advanced breast cancer survival	Hostility, guilt, negative affect 'Adjustment' Positive attitudes towards treatment	→ ← ←	SCL-90 ABS GAIS Structured interview
4. Rogentine *et al.* 1979	Melanoma progression	'Adjustment to illness'	→	Adjustment to illness Rating Scale (1–100)
5. Visintainer and Casey 1984	Melanoma progression	Problem minimization Anxiety, hostility NK cell activity	← → →	Ways of Coping Checklist SCL-90
6. Levy *et al.* 1985	Early stage breast cancer prognosis	'Adjustment' Listlessness, apathy Social support NK cell activity	← ← → →	GAIS POMS Interview subscale

Study	Topic	Variable		Method
7. Temoshok et al. 1985	Melanoma prognosis	Type C, younger Ss (cooperative, unassertive, suppresses negative emotions, complies with external authority)	←	Content analysis of videotaped interview subscale: Non-verbal Type C – 17 Semantic Differential Scales
8. Greer et al. 1985	Early stage breast cancer survival	Stoic Helpless	← ←	Categorical ratings of baseline interview content
9. Levy et al. 1986	Early stage breast cancer prognosis Predictors of NK activity on follow-up	'Adjustment' Listlessness, apathy Social support	← ← →	GAIS POMS Interview
10. Levy et al. 1986	Advanced breast cancer survival	Disease-free interval Joy Doctor's prognosis Number of metastatic sites	→ → → ←	Affect Balance Scale

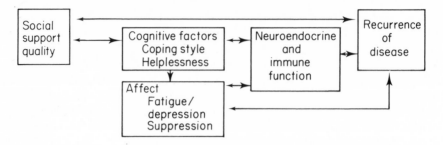

Figure 1: Prospective model.

social support, cognitively generated helplessness, and inadequate expression of negative emotion. Figure 1 displays a prospective model incorporating these factors. First we will address the factors individually, then the proposed interrelationships.

1. Social Support

Despite a relatively large literature, only a few investigators have studied the biological advantages accruing from social support (Berkman and Syme, 1979; Funch and Mettlin, 1982; Funch and Marshall, 1983); fewer still have considered possible links between this environmental interaction and possible biological mediating mechanisms. In our study of early stage breast cancer patients (Levy *et al.*, 1985, 1987), women who complained about a lack of social support in their home environment—for example a poor relationship with the spouse, decreased communication with family members and generally unsatisfying interactions with them—tended to have the worst prognosis. Perceived social support accounted for nearly 15 per cent of the variance in NK cell activity in this study. Recent epidemiological data (Reynolds and Kaplan, 1986) showed that women who had fewer social contacts, and who felt isolated, had a significantly greater risk of getting cancer (relative hazard = 1.7, $p < 0.05$), of dying from cancer (relative hazard = 2.5, $p < 0.005$) and of dying from malignancies at hormonally dependent sites (relative hazard = 4.8, $p < 0.01$), after controlling for other risk factors.

Social support research has been fraught with methodological difficulties. But we believe that the quality of perceived social support plays an important role in host vulnerability to stress and disease, and that this variable should be refined and incorporated into research in this area.

2. Cognitively Generated Helplessness

Behavioral helplessness induction in animal systems is associated with experimental tumor growth. Our pilot data reviewed above also indicated that helplessness in humans was linked to cancer outcome. In the 1978 cognitive reformulation of the learned helplessness construct (Abramson, Seligman and Teasdale, 1978), depression is considered the result of causal attributions reflecting the belief that negative events are due to some chronic characteristic within the person that will affect everything they do. Depression *per se* has not emerged as a clear predictor of worsened clinical outcome in studies to date, but some of the elements of depression, such as an apathetic/fatigue cluster, keep emerging in study results. It seems probable that the third element in our model helps to explain this discrepancy.

3. Inadequate Expression of Negative Emotion

In a recent review of this area, Cox and MacKay (1982) concluded that the inability to express emotion was a significant risk factor associated with cancer progression. Variously characterized as stoic (Greer *et al.*, 1985), type C behavior (Temoshok and Fox, 1984) and repressive/defensive coping (Jensen, 1984), such lack of negative emotional expression has been repeatedly associated with worse cancer outcome.

A dissociation between indices of distress and its expression has been demonstrated in a number of reports. A series of primate studies (Coe and Levine, 1981; Levine, Johnson and Gonzales, 1985) has shown a clear dissociation between overt distress behavior and biological markers of distress response in separated infants. And in our own breast cancer study (Levy *et al.*, 1985), endorsement of the cluster of fatigue symptoms, rather than overt distress, had a direct relationship to prognostic status and a positive correlation with depression, reflecting substantial shared variance.

Sklar and Anisman (1981) postulated that when an organism cannot, or does not, produce a coping response that is sufficient to alter a stress-producing environment, the effort aimed at homeostatic resolution taxes the organism. In our patient population, it appears that unexpressed distress may take a biological toll.

INTERRELATIONSHIPS: THE MODEL

We and others are finding the quality of social support to be of major importance in this population. Therefore, as depicted in Figure 1, we are postulating a causal role for perceived social support. Social support could operate cognitively, with other persons modelling and reinforcing active coping solutions during situational crises. Successful coping may enhance self-esteem and affect the causal attributions a person makes such that more credit is assumed for positive events and less blame is assumed for negative outcomes. Successful coping may reduce the physiological concomitants of stress, allowing neuroendocrine and immune functions to return to homeostatic balance. This balance might be protective in relation to disease outcome.

When social support results in more effective coping, such support might function to help the individual avoid the negative emotional and behavioral sequelae of failed coping experiences. Failure to cope successfully with stress often generates the helpless/depressed symptom cluster. Again these symptoms have been associated with neuroendocrinological and immunological changes with disease end-point significance.

Alternatively, such social factors could act on emotional expressiveness because one learns the acceptability of emotional expression at least in part from significant others in one's environment. Optimal social support may facilitate expression of distress in time of crisis, and also provide a higher likelihood that the distress will be dealt with and constructively resolved. This hypothesis is supported by the finding that adequate social support during a severe crisis provided the opportunity, welcomed by the victim, to express disturbance (Lehman, Wortman and Williams, 1984).

There are, of course, other mechanisms by which social support could interact with the emotional, behavioral and biological variables in our model. For example, support from others might also act directly through some other route—by enhancing compliance with a medical regimen, for example.

All of these possible pathways may have bidirectional effects. Cognitive helplessness and emotional distortion could certainly have a variety of effects on the social support system. Disease processes and endocrine levels can affect mood and behavior. And worsening disease course itself will probably affect social support. James, Mulaik and Brett (1982) have published a statistical method for testing directionality of association which might be of use in future research.

CONCLUDING REMARKS

We and others have found ample evidence that behavioral factors (including emotions and cognitions) are linked with disease outcome. The question is, if we change the behavior, can we change the disease course? Results of work in laboratory animals suggest that we can (Justice, 1985; Shavit *et al.*, 1984). But clinical trials and controlled experiments will be necessary to establish the causal link in humans. That process has already begun.

It is important to stress that the major determiners of cancer outcome are biological: tumor type, how far the cancer has progressed before treatment is begun, and the biological treatments available for such tumors. But for some cancers, if behavior matters—and we see evidence that it does—this is important because behaviors can be changed. Again, whether such change would affect the course of established disease is the next question to be answered.

REFERENCES

Abramson, L., Seligman, M., and Teasdale, J. (1978). Learned helplessness in humans: Critique and reformulation, *J. Abnorm. Psychol.*, **87**, 49–74.

Aoki, T., Usuda, T., Miyakoshi, H., Tamura, K., and Herberman, R. (unpublished manuscript). Low NK syndrome (LNKS): Clinical and immunologic features.

Beatson, G. (1986). On the treatment of inoperable cases of carcinoma of the mammary: Suggestions for a new method of treatment with illustrative cases, *Lancet*, **2**, 104–107.

Berkman, L., and Syme, L. (1979). Social networks, host resistance, and mortality: A nine-year follow-up study of Alameda County residents, *Am. J. Epidemiol.*, **2**, 186–204.

Besedovsky, H., Del Rey, A., Sorkin, E., and Dinarello, C. (1986). Immunoregulatory feedback between Interleukin-1 and glucocorticoid hormones, *Science*, **233**, 652–654.

Blalock, J. (1984). The immune system as a sensory organ, *J. Immunol.*, **132**, 1067–1070.

Bodurtha, A., Berkelhammer, J., Kim, Y., Laucius, J., and Mastrangelo, M. (1976). A clinical, histologic, and immunologic study of a case of metastatic malignant melanoma undergoing spontaneous remission, *Cancer*, **37**, 735–724.

Carey, T. (1982). Immunologic aspects of melanoma, *CRC Critical Reviews in Clin. Lab. Sci.*, **18**, 141–182.

Cochran, A. (1978). *Man, Cancer, and Immunity*, Academic Press, New York.

Coe, C., and Levine, S. (1981). Normal responses to mother–infant separation in nonhuman primates, in *Anxiety: New Research and Changing Concepts* (Eds D. Klein and J. Rabkin), Raven Press, New York, pp. 155–177.

Cox, T., and MacKay, C. (1982). Psychosocial factors and psychophysiological mechanisms in the etiology and development of cancers, *Soc. Sci. Med.*, **16**, 381–396.

Del Rey, A., Besedovsky, H., and Sorkin, E. (1984). Endogenous blood levels of corticosterone control the immunologic cell mass and B cell activity in mice, *J. Immunol.*, **133**, 572–575.

Derogatis, L. (1975). *The Affect Balance Scale*, Clinical Psychometric Research, Baltimore.

Derogatis, L. (1977). *Administration, Scoring, and Procedures Manual for the Affect Balance Scale*, Clinical Psychometric Research, Baltimore.

Derogatis, L., Abeloff, M., and Melisaratos, N. (1979). Psychological coping mechanisms and survival time in metastatic breast cancer. *J. Am. Med. Assoc.*, **242**, 1504–1509.

Funch, D., and Mettlin, C. (1982). The role of support in relation to recovery from breast surgery, *Soc. Sci. Med.*, **16**, 91.

Funch, D., and Marshall, J. (1983). The role of stress, social support and age in survival from breast cancer, *J. Psychosom. Res.*, **27**, 177–183.

Greer, S., Pettingale, K., Morris, T., and Haybiate, J. (1985). Mental attitudes to cancer: An additional prognostic factor, *Lancet*, March 30, 750.

Hanna, N. (1986). *In vivo* activities of NK cells against primary and metastatic tumors in experimental animals, in *Immunobiology of Natural Killer Cells* (Eds E. Lotzova and R. Herberman), CRC Press, Boca Raton, Florida.

Hanna, N., and Barton, R. (1981). Definitive evidence that natural killer (NK) cells inhibit experimental tumor metastasis *in vivo*, *J. Immunol.*, **127**, 1754–1758.

Hanna, N., and Fidler, I. (1980). Role of natural killer cells in the destruction of circulating tumor emboli, *J. Nat. Cancer Inst.*, **65**, 801–809.

Henderson, D., and Cannellos, G. (1980). Cancer of the breast: The past decade, Part I, *New Eng. J. Med.*, **302**, 17–30, 78–90.

Herberman, R., and Holden, H. (1978). Natural cell-mediated immunity, *Adv. Cancer Res.*, **27**, 305–377.

Herberman, R., and Ortaldo, J. (1981). Natural killer cells: Their role in defenses against disease, *Science*, **214**, 24–30.

Herberman, R., and Santoni, A. (1984). Regulation of natural killer cell activity, in *Biological Responses in Cancer*, Vol. 2 (Ed. E. Mihich), Plenum Publishing Company, New York.

Hersey, P., Edmond, J., and McCarthy, W. (1980). Tumor-related changes in natural killer cell activity in melanoma patients: Influence of stage of disease, tumor thickness, and age of patients, *Int. J. Cancer*, **25**, 187–194.

Humphrey, L., Singla, O., and Volence, F. (1980). Immunologic responsiveness of the breast cancer patient, *Cancer*, **86**, 893–898.

James, L., Mulaik, S., and Brett, J. (1982). *Causal Analysis: Assumptions, Models, and Data*, Sage Publications, Beverly Hills.

Jensen, M. (1984). Psychobiological factors in the prognosis and treatment of neoplastic disorders, PhD dissertation, Department of Psychology, Yale University.

Journal of Immunology (1985). **135**(2), August.

Justice, A. (1985). Review of the effects of stress on cancer in laboratory animals: Importance of time of stress application and type of tumor, *Psychol. Bull.*, **98**, 108–138.

Kadish, A., Doyle, A., Steinhauer, E., and Ghossein, N. (1981). Natural cytotoxicity and interferon production in human cancer: Deficient natural killer activity and normal interferon production in patients with advanced disease, *J. Immunol.*, **123**, 1817–1822.

Kalbfleisch, J., and Prentise, R. (1980). *The Statistical Analysis of Failure Time Data*, John Wiley & Sons, New York.

Karnofsky, D., and Burchenal, J. (1949). The clinical evaluation of chemotherapeutic agents in cancer, in *Evaluation of Chemotherapeutic Agents* (Ed. C. MacLead), Columbia University Press, New York.

Keys, H. M., Bakermeier, R. F., and Savlov, E. D. (1983). Breast cancer, in *Clinical Oncology for Medical Students and Physicians—A Multidisciplinary Approach* (sixth Edn) (Ed. P. Rubin), American Cancer Society.

Kikuchi, K., Ishii, Y., Veno, H., and Koshiba, H. (1976). Cell-mediated immunity involved in autochthonous tumor rejection in rats, *Ann. NY Acad. Sci.*, **276**, 188–206.

Lehman, D., Wortman, C., and Williams, A. (1984). Long-term effects of losing a spouse or child in a motor vehicle crash, Paper presented at the American Psychological Association Meeting, Toronto (August).

Levine, G., Johnson, D., and Gonzales, C. (1985). Behavioral and hormonal responses to separation in infant Rhesus monkeys and mothers, *Behav. Neurosci.*, **99**, 399–410.

Levy, S., Herberman, R., Lippman, M., and d'Angelo, T. (1987). Correlation of stress factors with sustained depression of natural killer cell activity and predicted prognosis in patients with breast cancer, *J. Clin. Oncol.*, **5**, 348–353.

Levy, S., Herberman, R., Maluish, A., Schlien, B., and Lippman, M. (1985). Prognostic risk assessment in primary breast cancer by behavioral and immunological parameters, *Health Psychol.*, **4**, 99–113.

Lewison, E. (1976). Spontaneous regression of breast cancer, *Nat. Cancer Inst. Monogr.*, **44**, 23.

Lippman, M. (1985). Can psychic factors transduced through the endocrine system alter the progression of human neoplasia? in *Behavior and Cancer* (Ed. S. Levy), Jossey-Bass, San Francisco.

Lotzova, E., and Herberman, R. (1986). *Immunobiology of Natural Killer Cells*, Vol. I, CRC Press, Boca Raton, Florida.

McNair, P., Lorr, M., and Droppleman, L. (1971). *EITS Manual for the Profile of Mood States*, Educational Testing Services, San Diego.

Moore, O., and Foote, F. (1949). The relatively favorable prognosis of medullary carcinoma, *Cancer*, **2**, 635–642.

Morrow, G., Chiarello, R., and Derogatis, L. (1978). A new scale for assessing patients' psychosocial adjustment to medical illness, *Psychol. Med.*, **8**, 605–610.

Morrow, G., Feldstein, M., Adler, L., Derogatis, L., Enelow, A., Gates, C., *et al.* (1981). Development of brief measures of psychosocial adjustment to medical illness applied to cancer patients, *Gen. Hosp. Psychiat.*, **3**, 79–88.

Nathanson, L. (1977). Immunology and immunotherapy of human breast cancer, *Cancer Immunol. Immunother.*, **2**, 209–224.

Papatestas, A., Paneviliwalla, D., Pertsemlides, D., Mulvihill, M., and Aufses, A. (1980). Association between estrogen receptors and weight in women with breast cancer, *J. Surg. Oncol.*, **13**, 177–180.

Pert, C., Ruff, M., Weber, R., and Herkendam, M. (1985). Neuropeptides and their receptors: A psychosomatic network, *J. Immunol.*, **135**, 820s–826s.

Peterson, C., and Seligman, M. (unpublished manuscript). Causal explanations as a risk factor for depression: Theory and evidence.

Pross, H. (1986). The involvement of natural killer cells in human malignant disease, in *Immunobiology of Natural Killer Cells* (Eds E. Lotzova and R. Herberman), CRC Press, Boca Raton, Florida.

Pross, H., and Baines, M. (1976). Spontaneous human lymphocyte-mediated cytotoxicity against tumour target cells. I. The effect of malignant disease, *Int. J. Cancer*, **18**, 593–604.

Reif, A., and Mitchell, M. (Eds) (1985). *Immunity to Cancer*, Academic Press, New York.

Reynolds, P., and Kaplan, G. (1986). Social connections and cancer: A prospective study of Alameda County residents, Paper presented at the Society of Behavioral Medicine Meeting, March 5–7, San Francisco.

Shavit, J., Lewis, J., Terman, G., Gale, R., and Liebeskind, J. (1984). Opioid peptides mediate the suppressive effect of stress on natural killer cell cytotoxicity, *Science*, **223**, 188–190.

Shimakowara, I., Imamura, M., Yamanaka, N., Ishii, Y., and Kikuchi, K. (1982). Identification of lymphocyte subpopulations in human breast cancer tissue and its significance, *Cancer*, **49**, 1456–1464.

Sklar, L., and Anisman, H. (1981). Stress and cancer, *Psychol. Bull.*, **89**, 369–406.

Spielberger, C., Jacobs, G., Crane, R., Russell, S., Barker, L., Johnson, E., Knight, J., and Marks, E. (1979). *Preliminary Manual for the State–Trait Personality Inventory (STPI)*, University of South Florida Hanson Research Institute, Tampa.

Steinhauer, E., Doyle, A., Reed, J., and Kadish, A. (1982). Defective natural cytotoxicity in patients with cancer: Normal number of effector cells but decreased recycling capacity in patients with advanced disease, *J. Immunol.*, **129**, 2255–2259.

Stoll, B. (1979). *Mind and Cancer Prognosis*, John Wiley & Sons, New York.

Strayer, D., Carter, W., and Brodsky, I. (unpublished manuscript). Familial occurrence of breast cancer as associated with reduced natural killer cytotoxicity.

Strayer, D., Carter, W., Mayberry, S., Pequignot, E., and Brodsky, I. (1984). Low natural cytotoxicity of peripheral and mononuclear cells in individuals with high family incidences of cancer, *Cancer Res.*, **44**, 320–324.

Temoshok, L., and Fox, B. (1984). Coping styles and other psychosocial factors related to medical status and to prognosis in patients with cutaneous malignant melanoma, in *Impact of Psychoendocrine Systems in Cancer and Immunity* (Eds B. Fox and B. Newberry), C. J. Hogrefe, New York.

Stress and Breast Cancer
Edited by C. L. Cooper
© 1988 John Wiley & Sons Ltd

Chapter 5
Psychosocial Factors Influencing Health Development in Breast Cancer and Mastopathia: A General Systems Study

Michael Wirsching*, Werner Georg, Florian Hoffmann, Jürgen Riehl and **Peter Schmidt**
University of Giessen, West Germany

INTRODUCTION—A GENERAL SYSTEMS VIEW

The question whether psychosocial stress factors have, in addition to biological factors, any importance in the manifestation and prognosis of breast cancer is very difficult to investigate. From a systems point of view, it appears quite obvious that certain inherited or acquired predispositions interact with situational factors in the development of clinical symptoms. To develop this further, it appears logical that the same factors which are responsible for the onset of the disease will continue to be of importance for the patient's further progress. Preexisting biological, psychological or social determinants will gain increased importance after a treatment has started, being either the source of additional negative processes or a positive resource in the attempt to overcome the disease physically, emotionally and socially. And finally, the disease itself becomes a starting point for another category of processes influencing the patient's (and the family's) future life, positively or negatively. From a preventive point of view, every severe physical illness carries a high risk of future biopsychosocial problems. Thus, every patient's situation appears unique and complex in its actual (here and now) and its historical (pre- and post) features. Circular interactions take place within and between the different subsystems (body, mind, family, etc.). Not homeostasis, but permanent change, ongoing development, resulting from

*Address for correspondence: Prof. Dr med. Michael Wirsching, Center of Psychosomatic Medicine, University of Giessen, Friedrichstrasse 28 D 6300 Giessen, Federal Republic of Germany.

continuous self-organization (autopoiesis) of the system, is to be expected. Any generalizing, static approach such as the 'cancer-prone personality' or a cross-sectional design appears highly questionable. The same critique applies in regard to a prospective approach, trying to predict what is the result of a *qualitative* change. From a systems point of view, the result of self-organization will hardly be predictable. And finally, our accustomed therapeutic strategy needs to be questioned. Instead of 'rehabilitating' the patient by strengthening social support, improving coping strategies or improving the quality of life, the patient's physical, emotional and social potential for development should be strengthened, to create the individually appropriate solution for the respective 'illness dilemma'.

Starting from this general systems point of view, we will now proceed to reduce this initial complexity, to draw conclusions which until now have all too often been neglected both in research and treatment equally. For example, rather than comparing breast cancer patients with 'normals' and 'controls', we will examine the *same* psychosocial processes operating in certain breast cancer patients, as well as in certain individuals living in the general population. As a starting point, we can choose the same stressful life situation: women awaiting a breast biopsy. In this initial distressing situation, we can expect to perceive most clearly those coping processes which the patient has probably used in the past and will most probably use in the future to overcome psychosocial stress. We can further assume that different coping strategies are of different quality as far as the maintenance of the patient's developmental potential is concerned. Insufficient and inappropriate coping strategies, and existing stressful life situations, will result in a negative outcome. Such patients are believed to be more prone to psychological and physiological disorders. They will have the poorest cancer prognosis, highest rates of additional diseases (mental and physical) and highest death rates. As a basic feature of a systems analysis, we will draw our variables from biological data, psychological factors (e.g. coping) and family assessment (social support, life situation and illness behaviour). A long-term (five years) follow-up will show whether certain factors have an unfavorable impact on women who either suffer from breast cancer or have a benign breast lesion, both having been assessed in the same medical situation the day before a biopsy.

SPECIFIC PERSONALITY PROFILE, PRIMARY PSYCHOSOMATIC FACTORS OR COPING MECHANISMS

Mammary carcinoma is the most intensively studied form of cancer in regard to psychosocial stress. The early studies of Bacon, Renneker and Cutler (1952) at the Chicago Institute of Psychoanalysis provided a list of characteristics which has been only slightly modified in later studies. In addition, the 'specificity concept' as developed by the Chicago school (Alexander, 1971) and characteristic of psychosomatic medicine in the 1950s and 1960s was also promulgated, that is, that certain personality profiles lead to specific diseases. In the 1970s, it became apparent that the most often mentioned influences—suppression of stressful emotions, rationalization, avoidance of conflict and overaccommodation—could be understood, in the sense of 'primary psychosomatic factors' (Alexithymia, Nemiah and Sifneos, 1970) or *pensée opératoire* (Marty, De M'Uzan and David, 1963), as an expression and consequence of an inadequate attempt to master one's helplessness and hopelessness (Schmale and Iker, 1971). This suggests that we are not simply dealing here with the various components of a psychosomatic personality structure, but rather with an attempt by the individual to be in command of the emotional stresses which occur in all serious and chronic diseases.

The concept of coping has received much attention in the field of psychosomatic medicine in the 1980s. It appears that one's coping strategy and premorbid personality are strongly linked, to some extent in a pathogenetic manner, that is, that inadequate attempts to resolve conflicts (for instance by avoidance) over extended periods of time become sources of new stresses. The question of whether psychosomatic factors promote breast cancer can only be clarified (if at all) by long-term prospective studies. More readily observable, however, are other manifestations of the general pathogenetic system: the individual manner of coping with the disease and the biological course of the disease after diagnosis. We have placed these two aspects and their interrelationships in the forefront of our own studies.

FORMULATION OF THE PROBLEM AND HYPOTHESIS

We began with the assumption that constant personality factors or communication strategies would be clearly demonstrated under the stress of the first diagnosis and the shock of the physician's information. We therefore examined women on the day before removal of a suspicious mammary node. This widespread prebioptic research setting presents great difficulties when a retrospective attempt is made to obtain information about the genesis of the disease. On the other hand, the situation is well suited to the examination of psychological/coping mechanisms in an early stage of the disease. In this way we have gained a foothold (same diagnostic stage and same examination stage) in the study of the clinically important question of to what extent various coping mechanisms are correlated to various developments in health.

The following hypothesis, which has intentionally been kept very unspecific, was the focus of the present study:

In addition to the patient's age, diagnosis (malignant/non-malignant) and developmental stage of the disease, psychological processes exert an influence on the general state of health over a long term (five years) following a breast tissue biopsy.

We report here on a descriptive screening attempt (pilot study) which, because of the limited number of cases, can only provide very preliminary results. These results, however, may help to serve as prerequisites for the generation of specific hypotheses and the formulation of complex working models in the future.

PATIENTS AND METHODS

Within the framework of the hospital's psychosocial consultation–liaison service, 62 randomly selected women were examined. The patients had all been admitted to the Department of Surgery (University of Heidelberg) in 1978 and 1979 with suspicion of breast cancer (Table 1).

Table 1 Research programme

T_1	1 day	t_2	5 years	T_3
$N = 62$		$N = 56^*$		$N = 52†$
Interview		*Bioptical diagnoses*		*Course of health*
Rating by interviewer and		Mastopathia, $N = 37$		Interview
independent judge		Carcinoma *in situ*, $N = 7$		Hospital charts
Content analysis		Carcinoma (T×N×Mo),		Family doctors
(Gottschalk–Gleser)		$N = 12$		
Questionnaire				
PSS16K				
(96 items, 16 scales)				
Rationalization				
(Grossarth-Maticek				
15 items, 1 scale)				

*Six women were excluded from the original sample for not fulfilling the research criterion (metastases or other malignancies). In one patient who had been diagnosed 'benign' originally later detailed histological analysis revealed a carcinoma *in situ*. There is thus a numerical difference to the previously published figures (Wirsching *et al.*, 1982, 1985).
†For four women no follow-up data were obtained.

The basis for test evaluation was an interview between patient and respective counseling physician one day before the biopsy. In addition, a questionnaire was instrumented, which the women filled out immediately after the interview and before the operation. Evaluation of the interview was by content analysis, developed by Gottschalk and Gleser, and, in addition, by means of a rating system developed by our research group especially for this study (ten items, each with a seven-point scale).* Each interview was evaluated twice by the respective consultant (two men and one woman), as

*In the evaluation which follows we used a recoded version with a scale of five. The rare extreme values were taken together (1 or 2 = 1 and 6 or 7 = 5).

well as by an independent judge, the latter having only a tape recording, from which all medical information had been erased.

As a questionnaire, we chose the PSS 16K, an abridged version of PSS 25 (96 items on sixteen different scales), which had been validated by Hehl and Hehl (1975) for psychosomatic characteristics, in particular for heart attack patients.* In addition, fifteen questions provided by Grossarth-Matticek were included. These latter questions have been shown to be valid in a prospective study (Grossarth-Maticek, Jankovic and Vetter, 1982) for the prediction of a malignant disease.

The results of the prebioptic studies have already been published elsewhere (Wirsching *et al.*, 1982, 1985). In a five-year follow-up based upon patient interviews, clinical data and data from attending physicians, a complete picture could be obtained of further developments in the state of health of 52 out of 60 cases.†

In the five-year follow-up study, nineteen women with malignancies are compared to 33 women who had benign biopsy results. The cancer patients have an average age of 59.8 (41–76) years, notably older than the comparison group, with 47.2 (24–70) years. Therefore the influence of age was especially considered in further evaluations.

RESULTS OF THE FIVE-YEAR FOLLOW-UP STUDY

Five years after the sample biopsy, the following picture was obtained for the course of health of the various patients in the intervening time (Table 2).

Table 2. Five-Year Follow-Up—Course of Health

State of health	Carcinoma ($N = 19$)	Mastopathy ($N = 33$)
Healthy	6	21
Worsened	7	10
Dead	6	2

One third of the breast cancer patients showed a stable condition, i.e. they had neither a recurrence of the tumor nor any other serious illness. In another third of this group, the general health condition had worsened due to serious illness in the intervening time (four tumor recurrences). The last

*In the interim this test has been published in a final version as *Psychosomatischer Einstellungsfragebogen*—PEF (Hehl and Wirsching, 1983).
†Of 62 patients, six were eliminated immediately after biopsy either because the cancer was in an advanced stage (metastasis) or because the women had previously had breast, or another form of, cancer. For four patients it was not possible to obtain data on the further course of the disease.

third had died (all but one due to breast cancer). In the comparison group, where the biopsies had all shown a mastopathia fibrocystica, the prognosis is, naturally, more optimistic. Here, 64 per cent remained in good health, 30 per cent suffered a serious disease (one breast cancer) and two patients died (one of gastrocarcinoma, the other after cholecystectomy).

By means of multiple regression, we have studied the influences which affected the health of the 52 patients in the five years after biopsy. As a first step we applied various regression models to the age and diagnosis (mastopathy—carcinoma *in situ*—T×N×Mo), together with only one of the instruments for psychological evaluation. In this way, we obtained a limited number of psychological variables which might influence conditions of health. The probability of error in this step was maintained at a 5 per cent level for the partialized influence on the target variable (beta weight).

The instrument which yielded the most satisfactory results was that of blind evaluation of the tape recordings on ten variables, of which four went into the model, with beta weights which occasionally equalled the influence of the clinical diagnosis. None of fifteen items in the Rationalization Questionnaire (Grossarth-Maticek) satisfied the selection criteria ($p < 0.05$). The Gottschalk–Gleser method (content analysis of the first ten minutes of the interview) provided no usable data in this study. Of these ten variables, based on the patient's comments and reflecting fear, aggression and hope, none fit the respective regression model. Of the sixteen questionnaire scales (PSS 16K), only one satisfied the selection criterion ($p < 0.05$) in the regression model.

The final regression model was calculated on the basis of five psychological variables, in addition to the diagnosis and age of the patient (see Table 3). At this stage we again tolerated a probability of error of 5 per cent. Accordingly, only three out of the five listed rating variables and the questionnaire scale significantly predicted the course of the health of the follow-up patients. In addition, as would be expected, the clinical diagnosis carried the most weight. The age of the patient could not be shown to be a predictor of health.

The variance estimation (multiple r^2) of the model is high (53 per cent) and statistically significant ($p < 0.001$). The three rating variables and the diagnosis in combination with the age accounted for equal amounts of the total variance (multiple r^2), at 23 per cent and 22 per cent respectively. In contrast, the questionnaire yielded a much lower value (multiple $r^2 = 0.08$). If all five psychosocial variables are removed from the regression model, the loss of variance estimation rises to 31 per cent (see Table 3).

Individually, the conditions which reflected an unfavorable development in the health of a patient (i.e. serious illness, terminal disease or tumor recurrence) were as follows:

Table 3. Multiple regression model to predict the influence of the patient's age, clinical diagnosis (mastopathia, ca. *in situ*, T×N×Mo) and five psychosocial variables on the course of physical health (dead, sick, healthy) five years after a breast biopsy

Variable	Beta weight*	Significance
Family ties (Questionnaire PSS 16K)	0.32	0.02
Rationalization (rating, strong–weak)	0.35	0.05
Altruism (rating, strong–weak)	0.27	NS
Stress 1 year before biopsy (rating, strong–weak)	0.30	0.05
Helplessness (rating, strong–weak)	0.40	0.01
Age	0.09	NS
Clinical diagnosis	0.49	0.00

*The beta weight indicates strength and direction of direct causal effect of different independent variables on the (dependent) target variable (course of health).

Variance estimation of the total model = 53% (mult. r^2, $p < 0.001$).
Loss of variance estimation after removal of all psychosocial predictors = 31 per cent.

—The sample biopsy revealed a manifest, non-metastasizing *breast cancer* (T×N×Mo)
—The patient stated in the interview preceding the biopsy that she felt *helpless*
—The patient stated in the questionnaire that she was receiving *little support* from her family
—The patient characterized herself as '*rationalizing*'
—The patient stated in the interview before the biopsy that the years just prior had been very stressful (*great psychological stress*).

DISCUSSION AND CONCLUSIONS

When comparing the present results with the available literature, one immediately becomes aware of a lack of longitudinal studies performed with careful controls, a lack which strongly contrasts with the otherwise prolific literature on psychosomatic factors in breast cancer. Only four studies containing correlations of psychological factors and course of disease data can be considered for comparison.

Derogatis and Abeloff (1979) describe a one-year follow-up study of meta-stasizing breast cancer. From the responses to a questionnaire and according to the opinion of the respective physician, the survivors all seemed less 'well adjusted'. In a 20-year study, Funch and Marshall (1983) found that in the youngest and oldest groups of breast cancer patients (but not in the middle-age group of 46–60 years), psychosocial stress and social support had a greater effect on the survival time than did stage of tumor. A 2½–3-year follow-up study in Heidelberg (Becker, 1979) indicated that active patients with plans for the future, those with hope and those who were constructively aggressive had a more favorable prognosis.

Most closely comparable to our study is that of Greer's group (Greer, Morris and Pettingale, 1979), in which patients were also examined before the sample biopsy was taken. The five-year study, however, was only correlated with coping behavior at a three-month follow-up, a time at which the first stage of adjustment is completed and the prognosis is much clearer than before the biopsy. 'Active denial and fighting spirit' were shown to favorably influence the course of recovery.

Our present results supplement the available literature. The influence of psychosocial factors on physical health appears somewhat more probable. This is in accord with what many physicians feel, namely, a diagnosis of malignancy is the only decisive factor in whether the patient will remain healthy or will suffer a serious or even terminal illness. The daily life situation, coping strategies and psychosocial factors are also of great importance. It must be strongly emphasized that we are far from having scientific proof, but on the basis of the present data it cannot be ruled out that people who feel helpless and lost, who have no confidence in their power to cope with difficulties, are more prone to illness than those who are more self-confident and have a feeling of autonomic strength. This result is in agreement with the conclusions drawn by Engel and Schmale (1967) more than 20 years ago, as formulated in their helplessness/hopelessness concept. These founders of psychosomatic medicine demonstrated by clinical experience that persons who have 'given up' or *feel* 'given up' are in grave danger of becoming victims of severe or chronic physical disease. Hence, we are not dealing with a cancer-specific symptom, but rather with a generalized and non-specific factor for susceptibility to disease.

A similar situation applies with the next effect, the unfavorable influence of rationalizing behavior. Avoidance or suppression of emotional stresses and conflict, which arises by emphasizing reason and rationality, occupies a central position in the psychosomatic theories mentioned above (e.g. Nemiah and Sifneos, 1970). A logical correlation between this effect and the feeling of helplessness described above seems apparent. At first it would appear to be a valid attempt to cope with a desperate situation by trying to be reasonable, remain rational, suppress threatening emotions, not let anyone notice anything. On the other hand, it seems clear that this type of coping strategy also has its weaknesses. Isolation, increased conflict tension, difficulty in overcoming emotional stresses (i.e. loss) can all result from an affective, long-term anti-emotional attitude. In the sense of a negative vicious circle, short-term attempts to cope in a rational manner would appear to be coupled with a long-term destructive psychopathogenic influence. That which is meant to assure psychological survival in the moment of maximal stress, over a long term becomes a personality deficit, hindering development and increasing vulnerability. This last indication applies, in particular, to persons who, because of developmental difficulties, began at an early age to control their emotionality in order to protect themselves from conflicts with which they could not deal, thereby isolating themselves from their surroundings (e.g. family).

That brings the next psychosocial factor into focus: relationships within the family. It would seem plausible that women who attempt to overcome their feeling of helplessness by means of rational control are particularly endangered if they additionally feel they are not receiving support from their environment. It also seems plausible that helplessness and rationalization encourage withdrawal of the family. The family is also concerned in all cases of severe or chronic illness. Proponents of the 'social support' concept (Cobb, 1976) point out emphatically the compensating role of the social network in cases of serious personal stress. On the other hand, in the (so-called) field of family somatics (Weakland 1977), the illness-promoting effect of an entangled, conflict-laden relational system has been described (for an overview, see Campbell, 1986). Once again we come up against the dialectic of processes involved in overcoming illness and processes which promote disease as sketched out above. The presumption of such long-term, stressful, conflict developments is supported by the fourth and last indication: the prognosis was particularly unfavorable when the women questioned replied that the year *before* the diagnostic biopsy was very stressful. Naturally we are not considering an acute stressor a so-called disease-triggering event (i.e. loss) as described for colitis ulcerosa, which directly promotes the cancerous condition. Rather, we assume that the present breast cancer condition was preceded by a long latency period, perhaps exceeding a decade, during which the tumor grew until it achieved a size adequate to be diagnosed (Fournier *et al.*, 1980). We interpret this psychosocial stress effect in the years before the examination as an indication that the present symptoms of helplessness, rationalization and weak family ties are the expression and consequences of an extended 'conflict development', and not the result of a short-term reaction to the present stresses. The acute stress would seem, rather, to intensify an already present psychological pattern.

In closing, it should be noted that our strategy differs in one important respect from the other studies mentioned above. We have tried, even in this pilot study, to show that the same psychological factors which above and beyond the patient's age and stage of tumor development affect the course of disease in breast cancer also produce effects in control group patients with mastopathia. We make the assumption that the psychological processes mentioned above can also affect the course of other (non-malignant) diseases, whereas this provides no information about the conditions or origin of the respective disease.

The present pilot study could serve as a starting point for more extensive studies in which validated methods might be used to test more differentiated hypotheses. As shown in the rating, the clinical evaluation must be considered of greatest importance. It will be necessary to obtain a larger and more representative sample and, in particular, more accurate biological data, i.e. tumor stage and grade. Additionally, we would recommend the examination of potential psychophysiological connecting links (immunological and endocrinological parameters), in order to throw light on possible interactions between psychological and biological processes. For this purpose, a longitudinal, three or four points assessment, perhaps during a 'tumor aftercare' programme, would be desirable. Patients with other diseases should also be examined in the same manner, since the parameters described here are probably not just cancer-specific and certainly not just for breast cancer.

Two aims may be achieved through such extended studies: (1) to broaden knowledge about the interactions of the biological and psychological factors during the course of various diseases; and (2) to develop prognostic criteria which will help to clarify for which patients in which stage of their disease psychosocial interventions might be indicated.

REFERENCES

Alexander, F. (1950). *Psychosomatic Medicine*, Norton, New York.
Bacon, C. L., Renneker, R., and Cutler, M. (1952). A psychosomatic survey of cancer of the breast, *Psychosom. Med.*, **14**, 453–460.
Becker, H. (1979). Psychodynamic aspects of breast cancer. Differences in younger and older patients, *Psychother. Psychosom.*, **32**, 287.
Campbell, T. L. (1986). Family's impact on health: A critical review, *Family Systems Med.*, **4**, 135–191.
Cobb, S. (1976). Social support as a moderator of life stress, *Psychosom. Med.*, **38**, 300–314.
Derogatis, L. R., Abeloff, M. D., and Melisaratos, N. (1979). Psychological coping mechanisms and survival time in metastatic breast cancer, *JAMA*, **242**, 1504–1508.
Engel, G. L., and Schmale, A. (1967). Psychoanalytic theory of somatic disorders, *J. Am. Psychoanal. Assoc.*, **15**, 344–365.
Fournier, D.v., Weber, E., Hoeffken, W., Bauer, M., and Kubli, F. (1980). Growth rate of 147 mammary carcinomas, *Cancer*, **45**, 2198.
Funch, D. P., and Marshall, J. (1983). The role of stress, social support and age in survival from breast cancer, *J. Psychosom. Res.*, **27**, 77–83.
Greer, S., Morris, T., and Pettingale, K. W. (1979). Psychological response to breast cancer: Effect on outcome, *Lancet*, **2**, 785–787.
Grossarth-Maticek, R., Jankovic, M., and Vetter, H. (1982). Standard risk factors

for lung cancer, cardiac infarct, apoplexy, diabetes mellitus and their changes in psychosocial context, *Psychother. Psychosom.*, **37**, 13–21.

Hehl, F. J. and Hehl, R. (1975). *Persönlichkeits-sualen System 25*, Beltz, Weinbeim.

Hehl, F. J., and Wirsching, M. (1983). *Psychosomatischer Einstellungsfragebogen (PEF)*, Hogrefe, Göttingen, Toronto, Zürich.

Marty, P., De M'Uzan, M., and David, C. (1963). *L'investigation Psychosomatique*, Presses Universitaires, Paris.

Nemiah, J. C., and Sifneos, P. E. (1970). Psychosomatic illness: A problem in communication, *Psychother. Psychosom.*, **18**, 154–160.

Schmale, A. H., and Iker, H. (1971). Hopelessness as a predictor of cervical cancer, *Soc. Sci. Med.*, **5**, 95–100.

Weakland, J. H. (1977). Family somatics—a neglected edge, *Fam. Proc.*, **16**, 263–173.

Wirsching, M., Hoffmann, F., Stierlin, H., Weber, G., and Wirsching, B. (1985). Prebioptic psychological characteristics of breast cancer patients, *Psychother. Psychosom.*, **43**, 69–76.

Wirsching, M., Stierlin, H., Hoffmann, F., Weber, G., and Wirsching, B. (1982). Psychological identification of breast cancer patients before biopsy, *J. Psychosom. Res.*, **26**, 1–10.

Section Four
Biochemical Processes and Breast Cancer Growth

Chapter 6
Neuroendocrine and Psychoendocrine Influences on Breast Cancer Growth

Basil A. Stoll
Departments of Oncology, St Thomas' Hospital and Royal Free Hospital, London, UK

Both psychoendocrine and neuroendocrine influences have been suggested as possible factors in the development and growth of human breast cancer. Psychoendocrine influences have been especially investigated, because clinicians who are familiar with the ability of hormones to either stimulate or inhibit the growth of breast cancer suspect that stress-induced hormonal change may have a similar effect. With regard to neuroendocrine influences, there are many reports of abnormal hypothalamo-pituitary activity in patients with breast cancer, and it is well established that emotional stress can modify hypothalamic activity. The topic will be discussed under the following headings:

—Distinction between pre- and postmenopausal breast cancer
—Hypothalamic dysfunction and breast cancer growth
—Hypothalamic dysfunction and obesity
—Hypothalamic dysfunction and depressive illness
—Role of neuropeptides in brain activity
—Switch mechanisms in cancer growth
—Psychoendocrine sequelae of stress
—Psychoimmunological sequelae of stress

DISTINCTION BETWEEN PRE- AND POSTMENOPAUSAL BREAST CANCER

It needs to be emphasized that breast cancer manifesting in premenopausal women shows clear clinical differences from the disease in postmenopausal women. The two groups show disparate predisposing factors, geographical distribution, growth characteristics and response to hormonal manipulation

(Stoll, 1986). These differences suggest that breast cancer in the two age groups is likely to respond differently to neuroendocrine and psychoendocrine stimuli. The widespread epidemiological practice of considering the two groups together may partly explain why so many investigations on the relationship between stress and breast cancer growth produce inconclusive results.

The factors predisposing a woman to breast cancer differ in relative importance between the two age groups. Thus, for premenopausal breast cancer in Caucasian women, the strongest risk factors are a familial history of the disease in a first-degree relative, onset of menstrual activity at a relatively younger age, and first full-term pregnancy at a relatively older age. For postmenopausal women, on the other hand, the strongest risk factors are abnormal obesity and delayed onset of the menopause (Wynder, McCormack and Stellman, 1978; Cuzick, 1986).

Again, it has been noted for many years that while postmenopausal breast cancer is particularly common amongst Caucasian women, it is relatively rare among women in Japan, Taiwan, Mexico, Africa and the Philippines. Among these latter groups, the incidence of premenopausal breast cancer is also well below that among Caucasian women. Both pre- and postmenopausal breast cancer become more common when Japanese women emigrate to the USA, but only among second generation Japanese reared in a western environment (Buell, 1973). In postmenopausal women, the increased incidence is assumed to result from the change in diet and increased trend to obesity. But since adolescent Japanese/American girls show earlier onset of menstrual activity (presumably triggered by their higher weight when living in the USA), it may be the early onset of menstrual activity which increases the predisposition to premenopausal breast cancer.

Pre- and postmenopausal breast cancers not only have different risk factors, but also show different characteristics in their type of growth and pattern of spread (Stoll, 1986). They also respond differently to change in the hormonal environment of the tumour, whether it has occurred spontaneously or been induced by therapy. Thus, oestrogenic hormones may cause stimulation of tumour growth in premenopausal women but inhibition of tumour growth in postmenopausal women (Stoll, 1981).

One would therefore expect differences between the age groups in their response to stress-induced psycho- and neuroendocrine changes. This might explain why lumping the two groups together has led to conflicting reports on the influence of psychological factors either on predisposition to breast cancer or on its course. Moreover, the influence of psychological factors is likely to be less in the aged because both endocrine and immunological activity are relatively decreased in older women.

In view of the number of factors which can affect either predisposition to, or the prognosis of, breast cancer, it is essential to use multivariate analysis

(Cox, Laszlo and Freiman, 1979) when calculating the possible influence and relative strength of individual factors such as age groups. Univariate analysis can lead to erroneous conclusions.

HYPOTHALAMIC DYSFUNCTION AND BREAST CANCER GROWTH

Under experimental conditions, it is possible to show that various types of stress can modulate the growth or spread of cancer in laboratory animals (Peters and Mason, 1979). In the human, however, it is difficult to identify the contribution of stress because it is merely one of many factors influencing breast cancer growth, and clinicians assume that it would usually be swamped by stronger host or tumour influences. Only in extreme circumstances, such as overwhelming psychological stress causing profound immunological or endocrine changes (or the presence of an extremely hormone-sensitive cancer), would its influence become manifest clinically. Even then, the growth of advanced disease is less likely to be affected because of increased tumour aggressiveness and freedom from restraints in more advanced cancer (Stoll, 1982).

In assessing the relationship between emotional stress and the growth of breast cancer, it may be useful to distinguish between the role of stress in increasing susceptibility to cancer, its role in triggering clinical activity and its role in affecting the prognosis of existing cancer (Figure 1). The growth

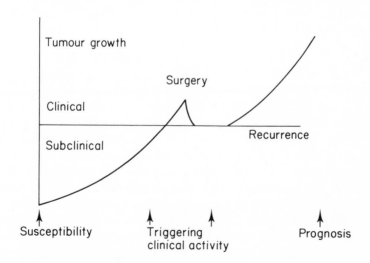

Figure 1: Possible areas for influence of stress on breast cancer growth (reproduced from Stoll (1981) by permission of Lloyd-Luke, London).

pattern of breast cancer shows remarkable diversity between patients, and even from time to time in the same patient (Stoll, 1982). This is thought to result from an unstable balance between the intrinsic aggressive potential of the tumour on the one hand and restraining immunological or endocrine factors on the other. Thus, breast cancer, both in younger and older women, can be caused to regress by manipulating circulating hormone levels or by blocking the access of certain stimulating hormones to the tumour cells. Breast cancer may also show spontaneous slowing of its growth rate as a result of physiological change in the hormonal balance in the body, for example at the time of the menopause.

The past 20 years has seen increasing interest in the relationship between emotional stress and the activity of biochemical transmitters in the brain which can influence the secretion of pituitary hormones. Most studies have been on biogenic amines such as catecholamines (e.g. dopamine, noradrenaline), serotonin and acetylcholine. In the last few years, there has also been an explosion of knowledge on how neurotransmitter activity is modulated by opioid peptides (e.g. endorphins) and other neuropeptides discussed in a later section of this chapter.

Biogenic amines and opioid peptides are found in all parts of the brain but their concentration is particularly high in the hypothalamus. It is now clear that emotion influences the release of pituitary hormones via the median eminence of the *anterior* hypothalamus. This receives stimuli from the frontal lobes of the brain and also from the limbic system, which is thought to control emotion of a more primitive type (Figure 2). The anterior hypothalamus then releases neurotransmitter agents which stimulate hormone-releasing factors acting on the anterior pituitary gland (Figure 3). In turn, this gland releases the various trophic hormones which can influence the growth of breast cancers of a hormone-sensitive type.

There are, however, also other pathways through which the hypothalamus may affect the growth of breast cancer. Emotional stimuli can also affect the *posterior* hypothalamus leading to the release of adrenaline or noradrenaline through the sympathetic nervous system. These could affect tumour spread either directly or through the immune system (Figure 4). Again, apart from controlling the secretion and release of pituitary hormones and catecholamines, the hypothalamus has been shown to influence the autonomic nervous system (including visceral regulation) and the general immune response. The hypothalamus is therefore the key to the majority of psychosomatic mechanisms which may influence the growth of breast cancer (Stein, Keller and Schleifer, 1979).

Trophic hormones secreted by the anterior pituitary gland could affect the growth of breast cancer by several different mechanisms. In the case of experimental tumours in animals, gonadotrophin, thyrotrophin, corticotro-

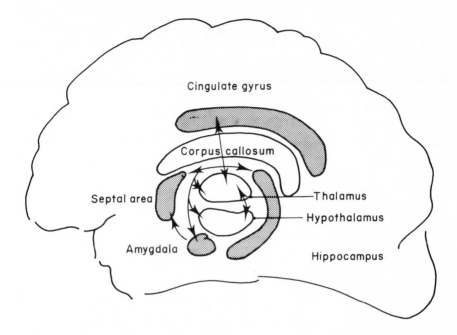

Figure 2: Interconnections of the limbic system in the human brain (reproduced from Stoll (1981) by permission of Lloyd-Luke, London).

phin, growth hormone and prolactin have all been shown to influence the development and growth of breast cancer. This may apply to the human tumour also, although it is gonadotrophin and corticotrophin (ACTH) which control the secretion of oestrogen, thought to be the hormone most directly involved in stimulating the growth of human breast cancer. Nevertheless, specific receptors for hormones such as progesterone, androgen, cortisol and prolactin have also been demonstrated in human breast cancer cells (Stoll, 1981).

Of the various mechanisms through which stress might affect the growth of breast cancer, the pituitary–adrenal axis has been subjected to most study. Whereas acute stress of the 'fight or flight' variety stimulates release of adrenaline, more sustained stress (such as that associated with mourning, separation, stress or anxiety) stimulates particularly the release of corticotrophin (ACTH) and cortisol. Stress may also stimulate the release of growth hormone, prolactin and thyroid hormone, while at the same time inhibiting the release of gonadotrophin (Curtis, 1979). But individuals differ so that the amount of cortisol release by stress varies widely from person to person and the release of one stress hormone may be independent of the release of another.

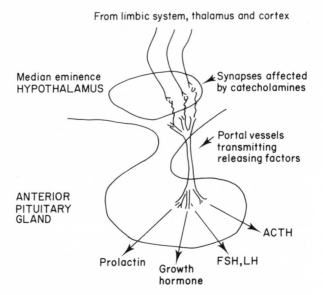

Figure 3: Pathways by which emotional stress may influence the release of anterior pituitary hormones (reproduced from Stoll (1981) by permission of Lloyd-Luke, London).

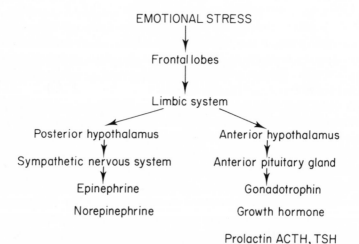

Figure 4: Possible mechanisms by which emotional stress may influence the growth of cancer. Effects may be mediated by either the anterior or posterior hypothalamus (reproduced from Stoll (1981) by permission of Lloyd-Luke, London).

Which of these endocrine effects of stress could affect the growth of breast cancer? A raised prolactin level may interact with oestrogen in promoting tumour growth, and an increased corticotrophin level may stimulate the secretion of oestrogen precursors from the adrenal cortex. There is evidence also that stress can cause depression of the patient's immune response (Solomon, Amkraut and Rubin, 1979) and this again might lead to increased growth of breast cancer. While cortisol is probably the major factor in depressing the immune response, both adrenaline and prostaglandins are also able to depress lymphocyte and macrophage activity. Finally, growth hormone and thyroid hormone may also play a part in modulating the immune response.

It appears then that several mechanisms exist whereby emotional stress and psychoendocrine factors acting through the hypothalamus might stimulate secretion of hormones which can affect the growth of hormone-sensitive cancer. *The mere existence of such pathways, however, does not prove that psychogenic factors actively influence the development or growth of cancer.* Clinical observations on the growth of the tumour in relation to emotional factors, together with parallel immunological and endocrinological studies, are required to prove such a relationship.

There are reports of increased corticosteroid production in breast cancer patients (Bulbrook, Hayward and Thomas, 1964). It was originally suspected to be evidence of adrenal dysfunction related to the origin of the disease, but the increased corticosteroid production probably results from the presence of cancer, as it is more marked with increasing spread of tumour (Durrant and Miller, 1973; Saez, 1974). Emotional stress will further increase the circulating cortisol level, and higher levels have indeed been found in breast cancer patients who appear apprehensive (Katz, Ackman and Rothwax, 1970). Increased excretion of corticosteroids in breast cancer patients may be associated with evidence of depression of the immune mechanism (Mackay *et al.*, 1971).

It is reported that hypothalamo-pituitary resistance to corticosteroid inhibition increases as cancer advances, and that those patients with a poor prognosis are especially likely to show impaired suppression of corticotrophin (ACTH) by corticosteroids (Saez, 1974). The relevance of this observation to prognosis is that in postmenopausal women, most of the circulating oestrogen is derived from adrenal androgens whose secretion is stimulated by corticotrophin. Impaired suppression of corticotrophin would therefore lead to higher levels of circulating oestrogen and possibly to stimulation of breast cancer activity (Figure 5).

The relation between hypothalamo-pituitary dysfunction and breast cancer is discussed in the following sections, particularly in relation to (a) the presence of obesity and (b) the association of depressive illness with breast cancer.

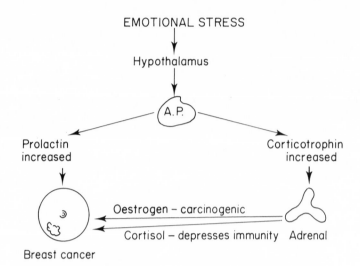

EMOTIONAL STRESS

Hypothalamus

A.P.

Prolactin
increased

Corticotrophin
increased

Oestrogen – carcinogenic

Cortisol – depresses immunity   Adrenal

Breast cancer

Figure 5: Possible effect of emotional stress on endocrine secretion in the breast cancer patient (reproduced from Stoll (1981) by permission of Lloyd-Luke, London).

HYPOTHALAMIC DYSFUNCTION AND OBESITY

There is considerable evidence that obesity is a major factor in predisposing women to breast cancer, both in pre- and postmenopausal age groups, but especially in the latter. A correlation between Quetelet's Index (weight/height^2) and increased risk of breast cancer has been shown in case control studies in Greece, Brazil, Holland and Slovenia (Miller, 1982). It is widely assumed that the abnormal obesity causes a higher level of circulating free oestrogen and that this is the factor which increases the risk of breast cancer in western women, in the same way that it increases the risk of endometrial cancer. However, the presently accepted view that the risk of breast cancer *results* from the obesity is not necessarily the explanation. Hypothalamic dysfunction is common among obese western women (Jung *et al.*, 1982) and this *could be the cause both of the obesity and of the increased predisposition to breast cancer.*

In support of such a hypothesis is the evidence that while increase in the size of fat deposits is associated with increased conversion of adrenal androgen metabolites to oestrogen, few reports confirm the presence of increased levels of circulating oestrogen in obese postmenopausal women. Again, in those cases where it does occur, one might expect it to be reversed by weight loss, yet this does not happen (Fishman, 1980). One might also expect to find increased levels of circulating oestrogen in abnormally obese premenopausal women, but again this is not the case (Zumoff *et al.*, 1981).

To explain these observations, it is claimed that even if total oestrogen levels are not found increased in obese women, they might still have higher levels of circulating *free* oestrogen because of the likelihood of subnormal levels of sex hormone binding globulin (Siiteri, Hammond and Nisker, 1981). However, the relationship between body weight and SHBG levels is one that varies considerably with race and environment (Wang and Allen, 1987).

Hypothalamic dysfunction may be a cause of obesity in postmenopausal women as shown by frequent signs of abnormal regulation of growth hormone, prolactin, insulin, glucocorticoids and sex steroids in obese women (Jung *et al.*, 1982). Hypothalamic dysfunction has also been suggested as the cause of the increased level of blood lipids often found in women with breast cancer, both in early and advanced disease (Beex, 1986). There is evidence also that breast cancer patients show a greater likelihood of hypothalamic dysfunction than do normal subjects of the same age and sex distribution (Schweppe, Jungman and Lewin, 1967; Bishop and Ross, 1970; Saez, 1971; Dilman, 1974). All these observations would support the hypothesis that hypothalamic dysfunction could lead both to obesity and to breast cancer in postmenopausal women.

A similar hypothesis might apply also to premenopausal women. Here again obesity is found to be a factor in increased risk of breast cancer, although statistically, the early onset of menstrual activity is a more important factor (Cuzick, 1986). In fact, the two risk factors may be interconnected in that girls who start menstrual activity earlier tend to be heavier, and their *adiposity persists through life* (Wang and Allen, 1987). A hypothalamic mechanism through which a critical weight triggers off menstruation is widely accepted, and an example of its effect on breast cancer susceptibility may be the increased incidence of breast cancer noted above in Japanese–American immigrants.

A link between obesity, hypothalamic dysfunction and premenopausal breast cancer has recently been shown in the polycystic ovary syndrome. In its fully developed form, it is characterized by abnormal obesity, hirsutism, elevated androgen levels and cessation of menstruation, and it is associated with a high risk of developing breast cancer. Its probable basis is hypothalamic dysfunction involving disturbed secretion of gonadotrophin from the pituitary (Zumoff *et al.*, 1983). Although relatively rare in its fully developed form, a less florid form is common in obese young women, where cessation of menstruation and elevated androgen levels are found to be related to hypothalamo-pituitary dysfunction (Glass *et al.*, 1981). Clinically unsuspected evidence of polycystic ovaries has been shown by ultrasound examination in 92 per cent of young women complaining of abnormal hirsutism (Adams, Polson and Franks, 1986).

These observations suggest that abnormal obesity in young women (especially when associated with hirsutism) may be evidence of hypothalamic dysfunction. In such cases, it may be associated with abnormal ovarian activity and increased levels of ovarian androgen secretion, and may also predispose to the subsequent development of breast cancer. This hypothesis is supported by the finding of ovarian stromal hyperplasia associated with *increased ovarian androgen* secretion in a high proportion of breast cancer patients (Sommers, 1955; Grattarola *et al.*, 1974).

The hypothesis does not conflict with the finding in a Channel Islands population of *subnormal adrenal androgen* secretion in premenopausal breast cancer patients, and also in women who subsequently develop the disease and in some of their unaffected sisters (Wang, Bulbrook and Hayward, 1975). No hypothalamic abnormality has been correlated with the finding, and the finding itself has not been confirmed in a USA report (Fishman *et al.*, 1979). This subnormal adrenal androgen secretion may distinguish a specific group of women with genetic susceptibility to breast cancer associated with adrenal enzyme abnormality (Zumoff, 1982).

The hypothesis is supported also by the finding in Japanese women of relatively low levels of androgen excretion and 'available' oestrogen in the blood (Hayward, Greenwood and Glober, 1978; Siiteri, Hammond and Nisker, 1981; Moore *et al.*, 1983). Since their susceptibility to breast cancer is much less than among women in the UK, it is unlikely that subnormal adrenal androgen secretion could be a risk factor for breast cancer in the vast majority of Caucasian women. For them, increased ovarian androgen secretion originating in hypothalamic dysfunction is more likely to be an important risk factor for breast cancer and this may explain the connection with obesity.

HYPOTHALAMIC DYSFUNCTION AND DEPRESSIVE ILLNESS

Clinical depression is found in about 20–30 per cent of breast cancer patients (Maguire *et al.*, 1978). Because depression often antedates the appearance of the cancer, it has been suggested that it may predispose to the development of malignant disease. The most impressive evidence is derived from the prospective study of Shekelle, Raynor and Ostfeld (1981), which showed the risk of subsequently developing cancer to be doubled in a group of patients found to be suffering from depression as assessed by MMPI testing. Although a cause-and-effect relationship has been suggested, it is more likely that *both conditions might be triggered off by changes in the activity of biogenic amines in the brain* involving both the limbic system and the hypothalamus. Some types of depressive illness are associated with reduced activity of brain amines such as noradrenaline, and it has been suggested that different forms of depressive illness may be based on reduced activity of different amines (Schleifer *et al.*, 1985).

There is evidence of hypothalamic dysfunction in about half of patients diagnosed as suffering from endogenous depression (Butler and Besser, 1968; Carroll and Davies, 1970; Schlesser, Winskur and Sherman, 1979). Cortico-steroid suppression of plasma cortisol levels and growth hormone response to hypoglycaemia have been the two most commonly used tests of hypothalamic dysfunction in such patients. Remission of the state of depression is usually paralleled by return to normal in the tests of hypothalamic function (Sacher *et al.*, 1973; Carroll, Greden and Feinberg, 1980). A neurotransmitter disturbance in common (e.g. serotonin or noradrenaline depletion) has been suggested for the association of endogenous depression and hypothalamic dysfunction (Carroll, Greden and Feinberg, 1980; Christensen *et al.*, 1980), the former representing neurotransmitter disturbance in the limbic system and the latter a similar change in the hypothalamus.

Another aspect of the relationship between clinical depression and breast cancer is the finding of a shorter expectation of life in patients who are apathetic and hopeless (Greer, Morris and Pettingale, 1979). While it is possible that apathy and depression themselves affect the prognosis, it is also possible that neurotransmitter disturbance in the brain may *result* from the presence of more active tumour (Stoll, 1981). Such a hypothesis is supported by the observation that the degree of hypothalamic dysfunction increases with increasing spread of breast cancer (Saez, 1974).

The mechanism by which breast cancer could affect neurotransmitter activity is not clear, but it has been suggested that cancer cells can stimulate production of an antibody which may block serotonin receptors in the brain. This could lead to the development of clinical evidence of depression and apathy (Brown and Paraskevas, 1982). It is also said that the depressed immunological reaction found commonly in patients with advanced cancer bears a striking resemblance to that seen in patients suffering from severe depression, whatever its cause (Schleifer *et al.*, 1985).

ROLE OF NEUROPEPTIDES IN BRAIN ACTIVITY

In recent years it has been found that virtually all the peptide hormones of the endocrine and neuroendocrine systems also exist in certain groups of central nervous system (CNS) neurons. The neuropeptides are potential chemical messengers in the CNS and include pituitary peptides (such as dynorphin, endorphin and enkephalin) and miscellaneous peptides (such as bombesin and neurotensin). Neuropeptides in the CNS may modulate the response of neurones to neurotransmitters such as monoamines, acetylcholine and catecholamines. They might be involved in several mechanisms which affect the course of breast cancer.

First, opioid peptides such as endorphins, enkephalins and dynorphins may exert an effect on behaviour, presumed to be mediated by the limbic and extrapyramidal system of the midbrain. It has been shown that opioid peptides are secreted by certain malignant tumours, and thus could be responsible for mood changes such as depression, which is not uncommon in cancer. Endorphins are also said to be released when patients resign themselves to death, and their secondary effect on the autonomic and neuro-endocrine system may be a factor leading patients to die earlier than would be anticipated from their physical status.

Second, there is evidence that endocrine manipulation, either by adminis-tration of endocrine agents or ablation of endocrine glands, can increase the number of opiate-binding sites in the central nervous system (Krieger and Martin, 1981). It is therefore possible that some of the pain relief following such treatment may be mediated by endogenous peptides, and indeed the relief of pain by acupuncture has been ascribed to such a mechanism.

Third, opioid peptides are released under conditions of stress and may play a part in modifying the growth rate of cancer. One possible mechanism is through their modulation of neuronal function in the hypothalamus, where they may influence release of pituitary hormones such as gonadotrophin, growth hormone, prolactin or thyrotrophin. With regard to corticotrophin (ACTH), opioids may either inhibit or stimulate its release depending on the type of stress (Grossman and Rees, 1983).

Finally, opioids may modify cancer growth through cell-mediated immuno-logical reactions to cancer involving monocytes, mast cells, lymphocytes and natural killer (NK) cells. It has been observed that endorphins can affect the activity of natural killer cells in man (Matthews *et al.*, 1983) and these are known to play an important part in the immunological defence against cancer. Nevertheless, the more important action of opioids on cancer growth is likely to be through the hypothalamo-pituitary axis, as described above.

SWITCH MECHANISMS IN CANCER GROWTH

It is important to examine recent evidence that the body is not merely a passive host to cancer but that the tissues react specifically to the threat of cancer growth and spread, and can sometimes modulate its course. In the past, it was assumed that such reactions were mainly immunological, but recent research shows that a switch mechanism involving a biochemical signal-ling pathway in the cell is commonly involved (Stoll, 1982). It has been shown that the relationship between malignant cells and their environment is an equilibrium which is readily disturbed so that reversion from a malignant to a non-malignant state is possible in certain circumstances and cancer cell proliferation can be stopped by local growth-inhibiting factors.

In the prolonged interval between the first genetic changes and the final appearance of cancerous cells, the stages to a fully developed malignant state may also be slowed up. Because the majority of established cancers show continuous and aggressive growth, some clinicians have deprecated the importance of such modulating effects by the host. Yet there are repeated clinical observations of fluctuation in growth rate, unexpectedly prolonged survival, prolonged dormancy or spontaneous regression in cancer. While controlling influences can be recognized only in a minority of patients, they occur in every type of cancer and are not necessarily confined to cancers showing an apparently slow growth pattern under the microscope (Dawson, Ferguson and Harrison, 1982).

It is now recognized that a cancer does not advance irrevocably at the same rate (Devitt, 1979). At different periods in the natural history of a cancer, growth may be rapid or slow, and in practically all experimental and human cancers there is a tendency for slowing of the growth rate as the tumour gets larger. In a patient with multiple secondary deposits at different sites they do not all grow at the same rate (Brennan, 1977), and different proliferation rates have been shown in different secondaries in the same patient (Willis, 1973).

The influence of host factors on breast cancer growth is most obviously seen in the spontaneous regression or slowing up of the tumour growth which often occurs at the time of the natural menopause. Similar regression, often of a dramatic nature, can be induced in hormone-sensitive breast cancers by hormonal manipulation, e.g. castration or treatment by anti-oestrogenic hormones (Stoll, 1979).

But there are also many cases where incompletely excised breast cancers never recur, or where secondary deposits lie dormant in the host tissues for up to 30 years before finally manifesting. Since dormant cancer may permit a very long lifespan and normal health, it is likely that in many patients death could occur in the interim from so-called 'natural causes', and the patient is, to all intents and purposes, 'cured' of the cancer. Dormant cancer is well recognized also in experimental animals, and in these the equilibrium can be easily disturbed either by immunosuppression (Eccles and Alexander, 1975) or by hormonal stimulation (Noble and Hoover, 1975).

Immunological or hormonal mechanisms have been assumed in human cancer mainly because these are the most common methods of regression noted in experimental cancers. The last few years have, however, shown that local growth factors (which may be produced by oncogenes) are the local mechanism deciding that a cell behaves in a malignant manner. Regulators of this type probably exist for every major type of body cell, although most evidence has been accumulated about epidermal growth factor, nerve growth factor, fibroblast growth factor, platelet growth factor and angiogenic growth factor.

Spontaneous shrinkage of cancer is real, even if uncommon, and does not necessarily involve complete and permanent disappearance of cancer in a patient. It refers to any measurable and confirmed shrinkage in the size of a tumour (primary or secondary) for a period of months or years, in the absence of treatment ordinarily regarded as being capable of inducing regression (Boyd, 1966). The recorded duration of spontaneous regression varies from a few months to over ten years, and in over half the total it lasts over two years.

Every year, between 20 and 30 new cases of spontaneous shrinkage of cancer are reported in the world literature, but the true incidence is likely to be many hundred times as large. The medical literature tends to record only dramatic cases involving large tumours. However, inhibiting influences are more effective when tumour deposits are small (and less autonomous) and this may explain why documented reports of spontaneous regression are relatively infrequent in breast cancer. Even if it were rare, the phenomenon of spontaneous regression offers proof of the reversibility of cancer growth, and enables us to study the phenomenon so that we might apply its mechanism in a larger proportion of cases.

It is now believed that both experimental and human cancers can produce growth factors which then act on their own cell receptors. This process maintains the growth of the cancer (Sporn and Todaro, 1980), and depriving the cells of these factors is likely to be a prominent treatment of cancer in the future. Specific tumour growth inhibitory factors have already been isolated (Todaro, Marquardt and Twardzik, 1982) and these appear to block the effects of specific growth-stimulating factors.

We noted above that spontaneous shrinkage of breast cancer is most commonly seen around the time of the menopause, presumably resulting from a switch in the local controlling mechanism following changes in the hormonal environment of the tumour. If physiological hormonal changes can induce tumour shrinkage by these switch mechanisms, could they not be also called into play by psychosomatic mechanisms? The likelihood is there, but it has proved difficult to identify the contribution of psychosomatic factors because of the multiplicity of factors which determine the progress of breast cancer.

PSYCHOENDOCRINE SEQUELAE OF STRESS

The previous sections have shown that psychoendocrine factors acting through the hypothalamus may stimulate release of hormones which are able to affect the growth of human breast cancer. They have also shown evidence of neuroendocrine abnormalities in certain groups of breast cancer patients and suggest that hypothalamo-pituitary dysfunction could underlie such abnormality. We still need to explore the psychoendocrine sequelae of acute and chronic stress.

Most of the classical data on the response of the endocrine system to stress are concerned with secretion from the adrenal cortex and medulla. Selye (1950) found that the ACTH–glucocorticoid system is activated in response to emotional tension and distress (and also to harmful physical stimuli), while Cannon (1953) showed that sympathetic activity is stimulated by acute emotions, muscular exertion, cold and pain. Subsequently, it was shown that the secretion of gonadotrophin, prolactin, growth hormone, thyroid hormone, insulin and glucagon can also be affected by physical or emotional stress (Curtis, 1979).

Acute stress stimulates the sympathetic system with consequent release of both adrenaline and noradrenaline. It is reported that noradrenaline released from sympathetic nerves is more predominant in mundane stresses (such as student examinations) while adrenaline released from the adrenal medulla is reserved for more acute situations of fright or flight (Robertson, Johnson and Robertson, 1979). It has been hypothesized that an abnormal balance between the two hormones may exist in emotionally inhibited individuals with psychosomatic imbalance (Taggart, Parkinson and Carruthers, 1972).

More prolonged stressful situations affect the release of hormones from the anterior pituitary gland, and release of ACTH will lead to increased cortisol output from the adrenal cortex. Various emotional states are associated with increased output of cortisol, for example mourning, separation, clinical depression and breakdown of psychological defences. Bahnson (1981) has suggested psychodynamic repression of emotion to be a feature of cancer patients, but most reports suggest that *conscious* suppression of emotion is a characteristic of people more likely to develop breast cancer (Greer, Morris and Pettingale, 1979). Is suppression of emotion likely to be associated with greater elevation of cortisol levels than repression of emotion? It is generally accepted that coping behaviour and anticipation of stress will decrease the adrenocortical response, but does an attitude of apathy and depression increase the response?

It must be taken into account also that cortisol is only one of the markers of the effect of stress on the psychoendocrine system. Stress stimulates also the secretion of growth hormone, prolactin and thyroid hormone, while the secretion of oestrogen, androgen and insulin tends to be suppressed. All of these hormones can exert an effect on breast cancer growth.

Growth hormone levels rise rapidly in response to exercise and emotion, but the response of growth hormone does not always run parallel to that of cortisol. Anticipation of a stressful experience may have a greater effect on growth hormone levels than the event itself (Kurokawa, Suematsu and Talmai, 1977), while repetition of the stress does not diminish growth hormone response as it does for cortisol. Prolactin levels also have been observed to increase in response to emotion and exercise, and, not surprisingly, a rise has been shown during sexual intercourse (Noel, Suh and Stone, 1972).

PSYCHOIMMUNOLOGICAL SEQUELAE OF STRESS

There is considerable evidence that emotion and stress may have transient effects on various parameters of immune response which are measured in cancer patients. These include changes in T lymphocyte response to mitogens, reduced secretion of immunoglobulins and reduction in numbers of helper T cells and natural killer cell activity. What is debatable, however, is the significance of these transient changes in host defence against human cancer. For example, T lymphocyte response to mitogens is significantly reduced after stress (Palmblad, 1981) and also after bereavement (Bartrop *et al.*, 1977; Schleifer, Keller and Camerino, 1983). This immunological change has been suggested as a possible factor leading to the increased mortality observed in spouses in the first year after bereavement, but similar changes are also seen in students at examination time (Baker, Irani and Byrom, 1985).

Possibly of greater significance is the observation that the level of natural killer (NK) cell activity is reduced after stressful life events (Locke, Hurst and Heisel, 1978). There is now considerable evidence that NK cells serve an important role in natural resistance against tumours and their spread. The activity of these cells is reduced in cancer patients, especially in those with advanced disease, and this observation has led to cancer treatment using stimulation by interferon and interleukin 2. In patients with breast cancer, cytotoxic agents cause a fall in NK cell activity (Brenner, Bennarosh and Margolese, 1986) and this may cause not only a decrease in immune competence against the tumour, but also against viral and other infections.

Corticotrophin (ACTH) and corticosteroids are generally regarded as the major endocrine mediators of stress-induced changes in the immune system because of their effects on B and T lymphocytes and on antibodies (Solomon, Amkraut and Rubin, 1979). Thus, Kiecolt-Glaser, Ricker and George (1983) have reported that some groups of psychiatric patients have increased blood cortisol levels and also relatively low natural killer cell and lymphocyte levels. However, pathways other than ACTH and corticosteroids may be just as important in immunological depression. Lymphocytes have been shown to possess specific receptors for catecholamines, prostaglandins, somatotrophic hormone, histamine and insulin (Melmon, Wainstein and Bourne, 1976) and normal macrophage activity is responsive to prostaglandins and catecholamines (Ignarro, 1977).

Other hormones also may play a part in psychoendocrine effects on immune function (Stein, Keller and Schleifer, 1979). The growth hormone response to stress is, surprisingly, dissociated from the corticoid response in that it may enhance the immune response (Gisler, 1974). Thyroid hormone also is involved in the modulation of immune function (Denckla, 1974) and its secretion responds to stress. Androgen levels in the male respond to stress and may have a suppressive effect on immune function (Wyle and Kent, 1977). Adrenaline and noradrenaline levels are increased in response to stress and will suppress various immune responses (Kram *et al.*, 1975).

There are also autonomic nerve connections with the thymus gland, spleen, lymph nodes and bone marrow which might affect the immune cells by releasing neurotransmitters such as acetylcholine, noradrenaline and endorphins. Specific receptors for these agents have been found in various immunologically competent blood cells such as lymphocytes, monocytes and mast cells. It has also been observed that endorphins can affect the activity of natural killer lymphocytes (Matthews *et al.*, 1983). While some endorphins stimulate NK cell activity, others suppress it.

Immunoglobulin levels in the blood have been related to personality (Pettingale, Greer and Tee, 1977). In patients subjected to biopsy for a breast lump, the mean serum level of immunoglobulin A was significantly higher in those patients who hahitually suppressed emotion, whether the breast lump turned out to be benign or malignant. A subsequent report (Pettingale *et al.*, 1981) showed that at three months after surgery, immunoglobulin M levels were higher in those patients who showed denial than in those who showed either a fighting spirit or stoic acceptance of the diagnosis of cancer. It has recently been suggested that some of the immunological responses described above may be non-specific, as they are seen also in association with severe depression from whatever cause (Schleifer *et al.*, 1985).

Recent research on slow-wave sleep (which is controlled by the thalamus) suggests another link between chemical activity in the brain and immunological defence mechanisms. Chemical factors closely related to serotonin are taken up not only by specific receptors in the thalamus (promoting sleep), but also by circulating macrophages in the blood (causing immunological activation) (Karnovsky, 1986). This may explain circadian fluctuations which have been observed in immune reactivity, and suggests also that disturbances in sleep patterns may be associated with disturbed immunological reactivity in cancer patients.

CONCLUSION

Long-continued emotional stress could be one of several factors influencing predisposition to human breast cancer or its growth rate. The influence is postulated to be through psychoendocrine or possibly through psychoimmunological mechanisms. Failure to prove such an effect in the past is due to (a) wide variation in the natural history of the disease between patients, (b) use of univariate analysis which ignores interaction between the multiple factors involved in either predisposition or prognosis, (c) failure to distinguish pre- from postmenopausal cases in analysis. They have different aetiological factors and may respond differently to stress-induced changes in the hormonal environment of the tumour.

The relationship between the growth of breast cancer and neurotransmitter activity in the brain is an important field for future research. There is evidence that hypothalamo-pituitary dysfunction may be a factor in predisposing Caucasian women to a high incidence of breast cancer. In the reverse direction, there is evidence that the presence of cancer may disturb neuropeptide concentrations in the brain, causing both mood change and also change in hypothalamic activity.

There is a mechanism by which stress might activate the growth of breast cancer, and on the other hand there is within each tumour a potential for spontaneous cure. As cancer progresses in the individual, selective forces lead to increasing predominance of more aggressive tumour clones, so that inhibiting influences are more effective earlier in the disease. This probably accounts for the infrequency of documented reports of spontaneous shrinkage of breast cancer.

REFERENCES

Adams, J., Polson, D. W., and Franks, S. (1986). Prevalence of polycystic ovaries in women with anovulation and idiopathic hirsutism, *Brit. Med. J.*, **293**, 355–59.

Bahnson, C. B. (1981). Stress and cancer: the state of the art (part 2), *Psychosomatics*, **22**, 207–20.

Baker, G. H. B., Irani, M. D., and Byrom, N. A. (1985). Stress, cortisol concentration and lymphocyte subpopulations, *Brit. Med. J.*, **290**, 1373.

Bartrop, R. W., Lazarus, L., Luckhurst, E., and Kilch, L. G. (1977). Depressed lymphocyte function after bereavement, *Lancet*, **1**, 834–36.

Beex, L. V. A. M. (1986). Metabolic diseases influencing prognosis, in *Breast Cancer—Treatment and Prognosis* (Ed. B. A. Stoll), Blackwell, London, pp. 200–211.

Bishop, M. C., and Ross, E. J. (1970). Adrenocortical activity in disseminated malignant disease in relation to prognosis, *Brit. J. Cancer*, **24**, 719–25.

Boyd, W. (1966). *Spontaneous Regression of Cancer*, C. C. Thomas, Springfield.

Brennan, M. J. (1977). Breast cancer research, *UICC Technical Report Series*, Vol. 27, UICC, Geneva, pp. 1–16.

Brenner, B. G., Bennarosh, S., and Margolese, R. G. (1986). Peripheral natural killer cell activity in human breast cancer patients, *Cancer*, **58**, 895–902.

Brown, J. H., and Paraskevas, F. (1982). Cancer and depression; an autoimmune disease? *Brit. J. Psychiat.*, **141**, 227–32.

Buell, P. (1973). Changing incidence of breast cancer in Japanese American women, *J. Nat. Cancer Inst.*, **51**, 1479–85.

Bulbrook, R. D., Hayward, J. L., and Thomas, B. S. (1964). The relation between the urinary 17-hydroxycorticosteroids and 11 deoxy 17 oxosteroids and the fate of patients after mastectomy, *Lancet*, **1**, 945–49.

Butler, P. U. P., and Besser, G. M. (1968). Pituitary adrenal function in severe depressive illness, *Lancet*, **1**, 1234–36.

Cannon, W. G. (1953). *Bodily Changes in Pain, Hunger, Fear and Rage*, Charles T. Branford Company, Boston.

Carroll, B. J., and Davies, B. (1970). Clinical association of 11 OHCS suppression and non-suppression in severe depressive illness, *Brit. Med. J.*, **1**, 789–91.

Carroll, B. J., Greden, J. F., and Feinberg, M. (1980). Neuroendocrine disturbance and the diagnosis and aetiology of endogenous depression, *Lancet*, **1**, 321–22.

Christensen, N. J., Vestegaard, P., Sorensen, T., Jarris, A. G., and Rafaelsen, O. J. (1980). Cerebrospinal fluid adrenaline in endogenous depression, *Lancet*, **1**, 722–25.

Cox, E. B., Laszlo, J., and Freiman, A. (1979). Classification of cancer patients, *J. Am. Med. Assoc.*, **242**, 2691–95.

Curtis, G. C. (1979). Psychoendocrine stress response; steroid and peptide hormones, in *Mind and Cancer Prognosis* (Ed. B. A. Stoll), John Wiley & Sons, Chichester, pp. 61–72.

Cuzick, J. (1986). Women at high risk of breast cancer, *Rev. Endocrine-Related Cancer*, **25**, 1–8.

Dawson, P. J., Ferguson, D. J., and Harrison, T. (1982). Pathologic findings of breast cancer cases surviving 25 years after radical mastectomy, *Cancer*, **50**, 2131–38.

Denckla, U. D. (1974). Role of the pituitary and thyroid glands in the decline of minimal oxygen consumption with age, *J. Clin. Invest.*, **53**, 572–76.

Devitt, J. E. (1979). Fluctuations in the growth rate of cancer, in *Mind and Cancer Prognosis* (Ed. B. A. Stoll), John Wiley & Sons, Chichester, pp. 9–18.

Dilman, V. (1974). Changes in hypothalamic sensitivity in ageing and cancer, in *Mammary Cancer and Neuroendocrine Therapy* (Ed. B. A. Stoll), Butterworths, London, pp. 197–228.

Durrant, J. A., and Miller, H. (1973). Non specific factors that may influence the significance of urinary steroid excretion in breast cancer, *Brit. Med. J.*, **4**, 767–69.

Eccles, S. A., and Alexander, P. (1975). Immunologically mediated restraint of latent tumour metastases, *Nature*, **257**, 52–56.

Fishman, J. (1980). Fatness, puberty and ovulation, *New Eng. J. Med.*, **303**, 42–46.

Fishman, J., Fukushima, D. K., O'Connor, J., and Lynch, H. T. (1979). Urinary estrogen glucuronides in women at risk for familial breast cancer, *Science*, **204**, 1089–91.

Gisler, R. H. (1974). Stress and the hormone regulation of the immune response in mice, *Psychother. Psychosom. Med. Psycho.*, **23**, 197–205.

Glass, A. R., Burman, K. D., Dahms, W. I., and Boehm, T. M. (1981). Endocrine function in human obesity, *Metalbolism*, **30**, 89–93.

Grattarola, R., Secreto, G., Recchione, C., and Castellini, W. (1974). Androgens in breast cancer, *Am. J. Obstet. Gynaecol.*, **118**, 173–79.

Greer, S., Morris, T., and Pettingale, J. K. W. (1979). Psychological response to breast cancer; effect on outcome, *Lancet*, **2**, 785–89.

Grossman, A., and Rees, L. H. (1983). The endocrinology of opioid peptides, *Brit. Med. Bull.*, **39**, 83–88.

Hayward, J. L., Greenwood, F. C., and Glober, G. (1978). Endocrine status in normal British, Japanese and Hawaiian Japanese women, *Europ. J. Cancer*, **14**, 1221–28.

Ignarro, J. L. (1977). Regulation of leucocytes, macrophages and platelets, quoted by G. F. Solomon, A. A. Amkraut and R. T. Rubin in *Mind and Cancer Prognosis* (Ed. B. A. Stoll), John Wiley & Sons, Chichester, pp. 73–84.

Jung, R. T., Campbell, R. G., James, W. P. T., and Callingham, B. A. (1982). Altered hypothalamic and sympathetic responses to hypoglycaemia in familial obesity, *Lancet*, **1**, 1043–45.

Karnovsky, M. L. (1986). Progress in sleep, *New Eng. J. Med.*, **315**, 1026–28.

Katz, J. L., Ackman, P., and Rothwax, Y. (1970). Psychoendocrine aspects of cancer of the breast, *Psychosom. Med.*, **32**, 1–17.

Kiecolt-Glaser, J. K., Ricker, D., and George, J. (1983). Urinary cortisol levels, cellular immunocompetency and loneliness in psychiatric in-patients, *Psychosom. Med.*, **46**, 15–23.

Kram, T., Bourne, H., Baibach, H., and Melman, K. (1975). Cutaneous immediate hypersensitivity in man, *J. Allergy Clin. Immunol.*, **56**, 387–89.

Krieger, D. T., and Martin, J. B. (1981). Brain peptides, *New Eng. J. Med.*, **304**, 876–85.

Kurokawa, M., Suematsu, H., and Talmai, H. (1977). Effect of emotional stress on human growth hormone secretion, *J. Psychosom. Res.*, **21**, 231–9.

Locke, S., Hurst, M., and Heisel, J. (1978). The influence of stress on the immune response, *Am. Psychosom. Soc.*, *Annual Meeting Proc.*

Mackay, W. D., Edwards, M. H., Bulbrook, R. D., and Wang, D. Y. (1971). Relation between plasma androgen sulphates and immune response in women with breast cancer, *Lancet*, **2**, 1001–3.

Maguire, G. P., Lee, E. G., Bevington, D. J., Kuchemann, C. S., Crabtree, R. J., and Cornell, C. E. (1978). Psychiatric problems in the first year after mastectomy, *Brit. Med. J.*, **1**, 963–65.

Matthews, P. M., Froelich, C. J., Sibbitt, W. L., and Bankhurst, A. D. (1983). Enhancement of natural cytotoxicity by β-endorphin, *J. Immunol.*, **130**, 1658–62.

Melmon, K. L., Wainstein, Y., and Bourne, H. R. (1976). Quoted by G. F. Solomon, A. A. Amkraut and R. T. Rubin, in *Mind and Cancer Prognosis* (Ed. B. A. Stoll), John Wiley – Sons, Chichester, pp. 73–84.

Miller, A. B. (1982). Obesity and cancer of endocrine target organs, *Rev. Endocrine Related Cancer*, **13**, 19–24.

Moore, J. W., Clarke, G. M. G., Takatani, O., Wakabayashi, Y., Hayward, J. L., and Bulbrook, R. D. (1983). Distribution of 17β-estradiol in the sera of normal British and Japanese women, *J. Nat. Cancer Inst.*, **71**, 749–54.

Noble, R. L., and Hoover, L. (1975). A classification of transplantable tumours in Nb rats controlled by oestrogen from dormancy to autonomy, *Cancer Res.*, **35**, 2935–44.

Noel, G. L., Suh, S. K., and Stone, J. G. (1972). Human prolactin and growth hormone release during surgery and other conditions of stress, *J. Clin. Endocrinol.*, **35**, 840–46.

Palmblad, J. (1981). Stress and immunologic competence; studies in man, in *Psychoneuroimmunology* (Ed. R. Ader), Academic Press, New York, pp. 229–57.

Peters, L. J., and Mason, K. A. (1979). Influence of stress on experimental cancer, in *Mind and Cancer Prognosis* (Ed. B. A. Stoll), John Wiley & Sons, Chichester, pp. 103–26.

Pettingale, K. W., Greer, S., and Tee, D. E. H. (1977). Serum IgA and emotional expression in breast cancer patients, *J. Psychosom. Res.*, **21**, 395–404.

Pettingale, K. W., Philalithis, A., Tee, D. E. H., and Greer, S. (1981). Biological correlates of psychological responses to breast cancer, *J. Psychosom. Res.*, **25**, 453–58.

Robertson, D., Johnson, D. A., and Robertson, R. M. (1979). Comparative assessment of stimuli that release neuronal and adrenomedullary catecholamines in man, *Circulation*, **59**, 637–43.

Sacher, E. J., Hellman, L., Roffwarg, H. P., Halpern, F. S., Fukushima, D. K., and Gallagher, T. F. (1973). Disrupted 24 hour pattern of cortisol secretion in psychotic depression, *Arch. Psychiat.*, **28**, 19–24.

Saez, S. (1971). Adrenal function in cancer: relation to the evolution, *Europ. J. Cancer*, **7**, 381–87.

Saez, S. (1974). Corticotrophin secretion in breast cancer, in *Mammary Cancer and Neuroendocrine Therapy* (Ed. B. A. Stoll), Butterworths, London, pp. 101–22.

Schleifer, S. J., Keller, S. E., and Camerino, M. (1983). Suppression of lymphocyte stimulation following bereavement, *J. Am. Med. Assoc.*, **250**, 374–77.

Schleifer, S. J., Keller, S. E., Siris, S. G., Davis, K. L., and Stein, M. (1985). Lymphocyte function in ambulatory depressed patients, hospitalised schizophrenic patients and patients hospitalised for herniorrhaphy, *Arch. Gen. Psychiat.*, **42**, 129–133.

Schlesser, M. A., Winskur, G., and Sherman, B. M. (1979). Genetic subtypes of unipolar primary depressive illness distinguished by hypothalamic pituitary adrenal axis activity, *Lancet*, **I**, 739–41.

Schweppe, J. S., Jungman, R. A., and Lewin, I. (1967). Urine steroid excretion in post-menopausal cancer of the breast, *Cancer*, **20**, 155–63.

Selye, H. (1950). *Stress*, ACTA, Montreal.

Shekelle, R. B., Raynor, W. J., and Ostfeld, A. M. (1981). Psychological depression and 17 year risk of death from cancer, *Psychosom. Med.*, **43**, 117–25.

Siiteri, P. K., Hammond, G. L., and Nisker, J. A. (1981). Increased availability of serum estrogens in breast cancer, in *Hormones and Breast Cancer* (Eds M. C. Pike and P. K. Siiteri), Cold Spring Harbor Laboratory, New York, pp. 87–101.

Solomon, G. F., Amkraut, A. A., and Rubin, R. T. (1979). Stress and psychoimmunological response, in *Mind and Cancer Prognosis* (Ed. B. A. Stoll), John Wiley & Sons, Chichester, pp. 73–84.

Sommers, S. C. (1955). Endocrine abnormalities in women with breast cancer, *Lab. Invest.*, **4**, 160–67.

Sporn, M. B., and Todaro, G. J. (1980). Autocrine secretion and malignant transformation of cells, *New Eng. J. Med.*, **303**, 878–80.

Stein, M., Keller, S., and Schleifer, S. (1979). Role of the hypothalamus in mediating stress effects on the immune system, in *Mind and Cancer Prognosis* (Ed. B. A. Stoll), John Wiley & Sons, Chichester, pp. 85–102.

Stoll, B. A. (1979). Restraint of growth and spontaneous regression of cancer, in *Mind and Cancer Prognosis* (Ed. B. A. Stoll), John Wiley & Sons, Chichester, pp. 19–30.

Stoll, B. A. (1981). Neuro- and psychoendocrine factors in cancer growth, in *Hormonal Management of Endocrine-Related Cancer* (Ed. B. A. Stoll), Lloyd Luke, London, pp. 194–204.

Stoll, B. A. (1982). Introductory discussion, in *Prolonged Arrest of Cancer* (Ed. B. A. Stoll), John Wiley & Sons, Chichester, pp. 1–8.

Stoll, B. A. (1986). Age group and cancer prognosis, in *Breast Cancer—Treatment and Prognosis* (Ed. B. A. Stoll), Blackwell, London, pp. 173–87.

Taggart, P., Parkinson, P., and Carruthers, M. (1972). Cardiac responses to thermal physical and emotional stress, *Brit. Med. J.*, **3**, 71–6.

Todaro, G. J., Marquardt, H., and Twardzik, D. R. (1982). Transforming growth factors produced by tumour cells, in *Tumor Cell Heterogeneity: Origins and Implications* (Eds A. H. Owens, D. S. Coffey and S. B. Baylin), Academic Press, New York, pp. 205–23.

Wang, D. Y., and Allen, D. S. (1987). Determinants of risk and endocrinology of breast cancer, *Rev. Endocrine Related Cancer*, **20** (Suppl.), 61–9.

Wang, D. Y., Bulbrook, R. D., and Hayward, J. L. (1975). Urinary and plasma androgens and their relation to familial risk of breast cancer, *Europ. J. Cancer*, **11**, 873–79.

Willis, R. A. (1973). *Spread of Tumours in the Human Body*, Butterworths, London.

Wyle, F. A., and Kent, J. R. (1977). Immunosuppression by sex steroid hormones, *Clin. Experientia Immunol.*, **27**, 407–11.

Wynder, E. L., McCormack, F. A., and Stellman, S. D. (1978). The epidemiology of breast cancer in 785 United States Caucasian women, *Cancer*, **41**, 2341–54.

Zumoff, B. (1982). Hormone profiles and the epidemiology of breast cancer, in *Endocrine Relationships in Breast Cancer* (Ed. B. A. Stoll), Heinemann Medical, London, pp. 3–23.

Zumoff, B., Freeman, R., Coupey, S., Saenger, P., Markowitz, M., and Kream, J. (1983). A chronobiologic abnormality in luteinising hormone secretion in teenage girls with polycystic ovary syndrome, *New Eng. J. Med.*, **309**, 1206–18.

Zumoff, B., Strain, G. W., Kream, J., O'Connor, J., Levin, J., and Fukushima, D. K. (1981). Obese young men have elevated plasma estrogen levels, but obese premenopausal women do not, *Metabolism*, **30**, 1011–23.

Section Five
Intervening and Coping with Stress in Breast Cancer Patients

Stress and Breast Cancer
Edited by C. L. Cooper
© 1988 John Wiley & Sons Ltd

Chapter 7
From Neglect to Support to Coping: the Evolution of Psychosocial Intervention for Cancer Patients

Alastair J. Cunningham
The Ontario Cancer Institute, Toronto, Canada

INTRODUCTION

Cancer tends to be viewed by our culture as a purely physical process, a view which has two unfortunate consequences. There is, first, a tendency to overlook the considerable evidence for an impact of psychological and social events on the development and course of the disease (reviewed by Cunningham, 1985). Secondly, the psychological distress that accompanies diagnosis of life-threatening illness tends to be downplayed. It is usual and understandable for health care professionals to be guided by the overt behavior and statements of patients, and to offer psychological, social or pharmacological help only when requested or when there is obvious deviation from normal coping patterns. This may be rationalized as a respect for the individual's privacy or as a necessary minimizing of costs, but clinical experience shows that many patients, although coping adequately, are privately anguished. The question for a humane society would seem to be: can this mental pain be eased, and do we value this relief enough to attempt to bring it about?

In recent years there has been a trend towards offering more systematic psychosocial therapeutic interventions to cancer patients. The main body of this chapter is a critical review of research studies on attempts to alleviate emotional distress in adult patients with cancer of the breast or other sites. The final section is speculative, and attempts to provoke debate by offering some unconventional ideas on possible new directions in this rapidly evolving field.

BASIC IDEAS ON PSYCHOSOCIAL ASPECTS OF CANCER

A number of features of the psychosocial impact of cancer seem fairly clear, both from clinical experience and from the literature (there is, however, room for debate and more detailed study on all the points made below).

1. Cancer often provokes distress

Emotional distress and social disruption often follow the diagnosis, medical treatment and progression of cancer (reviewed by Meyerowitz, 1980; Friedenbergs *et al.*, 1982; Petty and Noyes, 1981; Greer and Silberfarb, 1982; Telch and Telch, 1985). For example, Derogatis *et al.* (1983), in a multicentre collaborative project, found that 47 per cent of 215 randomly assessed cancer patients qualified for a DSM-III diagnosis, about two-thirds of these having adjustment disorders, typically with anxiety or depression as the central symptom. The proportion of patients considered to be so affected has varied greatly from study to study, probably in large part because of differences in diagnostic criteria. Many who are depressed may go undiagnosed (Petty and Noyes, 1981).

2. This distress can often be alleviated by psychological means

Evidence for this is reviewed below. It is worth noting that while it has often proved difficult to demonstrate, by objective criteria, an *average* benefit with groups of people, it is perfectly obvious clinically that many patients feel greatly helped by sympathetic interactions with health professionals and lay people.

3. There is a growing appreciation of importance of psychosocial health

Table 1 documents the increasing frequency of published articles on providing information and support to cancer patients. Measurement of 'quality of life' as a dependent variable has also become much more prevalent in the last 5–10 years (Holland and Rowland, 1981; Ware, 1984; Schipper *et al.*, 1984). This seems to reflect an increasing concern for patients' mental state while they are being treated for cancer.

4. Psychosocial interventions are evolving

Holland and Rowland (1981) have described the early history of this field. The period up to the 1960s may be loosely characterized as one of 'neglect'; while individual patients no doubt often received emotional support from family, physicians, nurses and others, there was little systematic attention to

Table 1. Frequency of published articles on psychosocial support for cancer patients over the last 20 years, listed by MEDLINE*

Subject of article	1968–72	1973–79	1980–86
Neoplasms generally	138 350	181 339	250 943
Psychological support to cancer patients	1	5	27
Behavioral/coping skills training for cancer patients	0	0	4

*Results of a MEDLINE computer abstracting search under the (pre-exploded) subject heading 'Neoplasms', together with a variety of key phrases on 'psychological' or 'group' 'support', 'intervention', 'therapy' or 'counselling'. Titles were printed out and scanned (by the author) for apparent relevance. The search was obviously not exhaustive and does not pretend to be accurate or comprehensive, merely to reflect an increase with time in psychosocial titles against a relatively stable and large background of general articles on cancer.

patients' needs on an institutional scale, in part because they were usually not informed of their diagnosis (Novack *et al.*, 1979). In the 1970s, systematic 'support' by health professionals became more common, as reflected in the beginnings of a literature on the subject (Table 1). In the last five years or so, as will be seen in the literature review below and in Table 1, reports on teaching ways of 'coping' with emotional problems have begun to emerge. (Instruction in overcoming the problems following specific operations has been available for a longer time.) Finally, the last few years have also seen claims for what we might call 'mastery' from psychosocial interventions, the radical idea that certain mental techniques might retard the physical disease, to which we will also briefly allude below. A progression seems to exist, from 'neglect' to 'support' to 'coping', with a possible future (and still largely unproven) evolution towards a degree of 'mastery'.

REVIEW OF STUDIES ON THE PSYCHOLOGICAL TREATMENT OF DISTRESS

1. Descriptive (non-experimental) accounts

Support groups for cancer patients, whether 'self-help' or professionally led, typically evolve locally to 'fill the gaps left by general health care' as Schwartz (1977) put it. Specific coping deficits are not targeted, but benefits to participants are mutual support, emotional ventilation, and problem-solving though peer discussion and modelling. Yalom and Greaves (1977) and Spiegel and Yalom (1978) described a discussion group conducted with a changing population of terminally ill patients over four years, dealing with 40 people in all: an ideal number of participating patients at any one time was considered to be seven. They concluded that the discussions were exceptionally therapeutic, major benefits being a chance to help one another, to express anger at their doctors and to talk about their dread and sense of loneliness at impending death. Dying was to some extent 'detoxified', and sense of meaning in life was enhanced. Ringler *et al.* (1981) have described some of the technicalities of conducting continuing groups, tracing the evolution of participants' attitudes from initial hesitation through conflict and struggles for domination to a greater group cohesiveness. They explain the need for leaders to define purpose and boundaries for the groups, to create a safe environment and allow patients to experience their sadness fully by demonstrating that the leader is prepared to hear about traumatic difficulties and pain. Obviously such long-term groups are expensive in terms of professional time, and are likely to remain available to very few patients. It is also evident that a subjective evaluation of their effectiveness by the group leaders is likely to be biassed.

Weisman and Worden (1976, 1977) make the point that not all patients need or want this kind of support, but that a majority of those at risk for psychological distress (about one-third in the estimation of Worden, 1983) will accept counselling (Worden and Weisman, 1980). Many descriptive accounts also express the general view that supportive groups and interventions are useful for cancer patients (e.g. Wood *et al.*, 1978; Capone *et al.*, 1979) as for people with other chronic diseases (e.g. Buchanan, 1978). Maguire *et al.* (1980) have documented the value of early detection and treatment of psychiatric symptoms among postmastectomy patients whose subsequent morbidity twelve months later was much reduced compared to untreated controls.

2. Experimental studies

The objective evaluation of psychological interventions for cancer patients is methodologically complex and difficult, as several authors have pointed out in their reviews of the literature (Watson, 1983; Friedenbergs *et al.*, 1981; Temoshok and Heller, 1984; Telch and Telch, 1985). Some of the problems are common to much psychotherapy outcome research: thus in many studies, incomplete details are given of patient accrual into and adherence to the treatment program, and descriptions of the intervention itself often lack details of the methods used, time taken, therapist qualifications and theoretical basis. Design deficiencies include the absence of any or of realistic control interventions, lack of randomization, and disregard for the probably important effects of patients' expectations. Evaluation of outcome may involve such obvious limitations as lack of follow-up or subjective assessments by the therapists themselves (open to bias), as well as more intractable difficulties such as finding truly appropriate instruments and deciding between self-reported or observer ratings; in this last case, while it may be argued that only the patient knows how he or she feels, there may, of course, be a reluctance or inability to express this because it seems socially undesirable or because the dysphoria is suppressed and unrecognized.

Other assessment problems are more specific to this patient population. The great heterogeneity of the disease is one of these problems: cancer is a mixture of many very different diseases, and even within one diagnostic category, e.g. 'metastatic breast cancer', there is great variation in the course of the illness. Apart from differences in diagnosis, stage of disease and medical treatment, it is also usually impossible to arrange for homogeneity in such important demographic variables as age, education, occupation and religious beliefs. An argument can be made (Telch and Telch, 1985) for accepting the increase in variance this uncontrollable heterogeneity entails, on the grounds that an intervention must be shown to be generally useful to a wide range of patients. Another problem arises from differences in people's adjustment to disease, suggesting that specifically tailored one-to-one interventions might be more effective than group therapy; there is little published work comparing them as yet. A third concern is that the instruments used for assessing mood disturbance vary from one study to another; they have usually been standardized on populations who are not physically ill, and may not be appropriate for cancer patients. For example, Koenig, Levine and Brenna (1967) pointed out that an elevated depression score on the MMPI could reflect realistic responses by a person with cancer to those items assessing somatic complaints.

(a) Supportive interventions

Bloom, Ross and Burnell (1978), using a non-randomized control group design, compared the affective responses and sense of personal control over events in women who had recently undergone surgery for breast cancer; 21 women received a psychosocial intervention, eighteen did not. This early report demonstrates some of the flaws discussed above. Thus the nature of the intervention was not clearly described, but apparently consisted mainly of brief, frequent individual visits by a volunteer or social worker while the patient was hospitalized. After discharge the patient was 'encouraged to use the services of an outreach centre', which included support groups, but there was no report on how many availed themselves of this, or on the behavior of women in the control group. Assessment with the Profile of Mood States (POMS) and Health Locus of Control (HLC) was at 4–7 days after surgery and approximately two months later. The POMS showed significantly higher affective distress on all but one dimension in the intervention group at 4–7 days: this was taken as evidence that the expression of negative affect had been encouraged (presumably in a therapeutic way), a conclusion which is not justified in the absence of preintervention data for the non-randomized groups. By two months, both groups scored the same on the POMS. HLC scores were the same at 4–7 days but significantly higher in the intervention group at two months, possibly indicating an enhanced sense of control.

A larger study, of similar design, was carried out by Gordon *et al.* (1980). Again, a non-equivalent control group design was employed, a total of approximately 300 patients with melanoma or breast or lung cancer being entered into intervention or control categories during different periods. Psychosocial intervention included education about living with the disease, counselling, and assistance with manipulating the medical environment. These services were provided by a team of health professionals, any one patient receiving care from the same counsellor throughout. The extent of contact varied, but averaged eleven periods of 20 minutes extending over six months. Assessment was by structured interviews and an extensive battery of behavioral surveys, plus psychological tests at time of hospital admission, discharge, and three and six months later. There was some evidence for significantly greater decline in negative affect in the intervention group, but differences were small and not consistent over time or for the three diagnostic categories. Self-report of problems and their severity did not improve with the intervention. The activity patterns of treated patients suggested more 'active' time use with a (non-significantly) greater tendency to return to work.

Linn, Linn and Harris (1982) conducted a study which also involved supportive counselling several times each week. Patients were seen by the same counsellor on an individual basis, but with more positive results than were achieved by Gordon *et al.* The subjects were 120 men with Stage IV (late stage) cancer; these men were randomly assigned to two equal groups, test and control (no intervention) being similar on demographic and medical criteria. Dependent variables included physician assessment of body impairment and activity plus patient responses to self-report questionnaires measuring depression (POMS depression scale), self-esteem, life satisfaction, alienation and locus of control. No differences were found between the groups in functional status or survival. Depression was significantly less at three months in the intervention group but not at the other times tested, one, six, nine and twelve months after entry. The other four self-report indicators all showed significantly better maintenance of quality of life, and in many instances its improvement, in the counselled group from three months right up to the twelve-month point, when only about 20 per cent remained alive.

Individual supportive and educational interactions were also used by Forester, Kornfeld and Fleiss (1985), working with patients who were receiving six weeks of radiotherapy for a variety of types of cancer. One hundred patients were randomly assigned to therapy or control groups, the test group receiving 30 minutes' intervention per week for ten weeks. Evaluation, at intervals up to fourteen weeks after the beginning of therapeutic contact, was by a structured interview carried out by an assessor who was said to be blind to the patients' treatment status (one wonders how this 'blindness' could be preserved in an interview of any depth!). The Schedule of Affective Disorders and Schizophrenia (SADS) was also filled out each time by the patient. It was found that dysphoric emotional symptoms decreased in both groups, but significantly more in the treated group; the improvement was greater for males than for female patients. Of great interest was the simultaneous decline in physical symptoms, anorexia, fatigue, nausea and vomiting.

There have been few attempts to assess objectively the effects of supportive therapy administered to *groups* of cancer patients. Spiegel, Bloom and Yalom (1981) randomly assigned 50 patients with metastatic breast carcinoma to a treatment category and 36 to a control (no treatment) category. Their report contains few details of the treatment, but there were apparently three distinct groups, each with two leaders, one of them a mental health professional. Patients remained in a group for up to a year, meeting for weekly 90-minute sessions; approximately one-half dropped out before this time, fifteen of the treatment group and eleven of the controls dying during the study. The intervention consisted mainly of the facilitation of supportive interaction, ventilation of emotions and discussion of common problems. Assessment was by self-report, at 0, 100, 200 and 300 days on the POMS, and measures of phobias, maladaptive coping, self-esteem, denial and perceived locus of control. There was no significant change in the last three of these indicators with time, while a significant decrease in fearfulness and maladaptive coping was found. The POMS showed that whereas the control category worsened steadily with time, the mood of patients in all support therapy groups improved, although a significant improvement over controls was not reached until the 300-day assessment. Slopes analysis demonstrated that the rate of change was significantly better in the intervention category, improvement being noted for all subscales except anger–hostility.

Jacobs *et al.* (1983) randomized 34 patients with Hodgkin's disease into a no-treatment control category or into a support group comprising eight weekly professionally led sessions of 1.5 hours. Assessment was by the Cancer Patient Behaviour Scale (CPBS), an investigator-designed and validated measure of mood and activity. At the end of the course there was improvement in some of the test subscales and worsening in others, but no significant difference between group participants and controls. By contrast, in a parallel study reported in the same paper, where Hodgkin's patients received bulletins of information about their disease over a three-month period, there was a significant improvement by the informed group compared with a randomized (no information) control in anxiety, depression, life disruption, treatment-related problems and knowledge of the disease. This beneficial effect of information simply given to the patients—there were apparently no group meetings—is a striking example of the therapeutic effects of knowledge at low cost. However, as Telch and Telch (1985) point out, the effects of information may prove to be encouraging to the patient when a disease, like Hodgkin's, is relatively responsive to medical treatment, but could have the reverse effect when prognoses are less favorable.

Other reports on the effects of support groups are either available only in abstract form or involve less well controlled comparisons. Golonka (1977, abstract) found no effects on self-reported anxiety when twelve group counselling sessions were given to nineteen breast cancer patients, by comparison with untreated controls (method of assignment not specified). Farash (1979, abstract) randomly assigned women after mastectomy to a self-help counselling group, individual crisis counselling or not treatment. Both kinds of therapy were said to be equally effective in alleviating body image disturbance and had some beneficial effect on depression scores, although no data were reported. Youssef (1984) found that a small group of eight hospitalized breast cancer patients receiving eighteen sessions of group crisis counselling showed significant improvement in self-esteem and depression ratings compared with a (non-randomly assigned) group of ten controls. Vachon *et al.* (1981), in a more comprehensive study with a quasi-experimental design, found that among breast cancer patients who experienced distress while undergoing radiation treatment, those living in a residential lodge with supportive therapy showed reduced levels compared with patients receiving similar medical treatment but no systematic support and living at home.

(b) Short-term, structured interventions

As in other areas of psychotherapy, there has been a recent trend towards use of more focussed short-term interventions in providing psychological assistance to cancer patients. The heightened awareness of the need for cost-effectiveness has also generally led to work with groups rather than individual therapy. There are, however, some accounts in the literature of the use of structured, behavioral interventions with individuals where objective assessment has been made. In a preliminary report, Tarrier and Maguire (1984) describe the application of a structured, 2–4 session, cognitive behavioural training program to women who were adapting poorly to a recent mastectomy. Ten such women were allocated randomly to one of two categories: those in the first received the therapy only, while those in the second received 'drugs' (Mianserin, an antidepressant medication) as well. The program was taught individually, and included relaxation training, anxiety monitoring, cognitive restructuring, use of positive imagery and behavioral practice. Both groups showed significant, large improvements in mood as assessed by the Beck Depression Inventory (BDI) and General Health Questionnaire (GHQ) at the end of intervention and at three-month follow-up; this was better maintained in the group also receiving drugs. In a similar study, published in abstract form (West, 1981), fourteen oncology patients with elevated BDI scores (>17) were randomized into two groups, the eight in the treatment category receiving eight sessions (apparently individual) of a cognitive problem-solving therapy. Most clients improved significantly over the treatment time, the mean reduction being 8.2 BDI units in the therapy group and 1.3 in the controls, a suggestive but not significant difference.

Weisman and Worden (1977) have thoroughly described the concerns and distress suffered by many cancer patients. As a natural outgrowth of this work they evaluated the effects of two kinds of individual psychotherapy: (1) a client-centered exploration of problems and encouraging of emotional expression, together with behavioral rehearsal and role-playing in some cases; (2) a more didactic skills-training approach to solving problems by breaking them into manageable steps, together with relaxation training (Weisman, Worden and Sobel, 1980; Worden and Weisman, 1984). The authors made a point of offering therapy only to the one-third of newly diagnosed patients judged at high risk for subsequent distress by the POMS and a clinician rating scale. Patients ($N=59$) were randomized into the two treatment categories and were seen individually once a week for four weeks. Randomized controls were not used because of the authors' concern that all high-risk patients should be treated; instead, comparisons were drawn with 58 patients classified as high risk in the early, purely descriptive work, who had a similar range of neoplasms. Assessments were done at intervals for twelve months using the POMS plus several author-constructed and validated measures of dysphoric mood; these showed a small, well-maintained decrease in emotional distress, the two treatment groups being indistinguishable and both significantly better than controls.

Perhaps the best evidence for efficacy and feasibility of psychological intervention in alleviating distress among cancer patients comes from controlled studies, most of them recent, on the use of short-term, structured, group programs. These are 'cognitive behavioral' in the sense of aspiring to modify patients' reactions to events by imparting control-enhancing information and teaching cognitive coping strategies. No doubt all of these groups also provided some support and varying opportunities for emotional expression.

The programme evaluated by Ferlic, Goldman and Kennedy (1979) consisted of six sessions of 1.5 hours conducted over two weeks with small groups of patients, most of whom had recently diagnosed, advanced cancer. Two professional co-leaders transmitted medical, social and spiritual information which was then discussed by the group. A comparison was drawn between 30 group participants and 30 similar controls matched for age, sex and education but apparently not randomly assigned (the report is unclear on this point). Assessment was done before and after the groups, and at six months, by means of an investigator-developed 'patient perception' questionnaire and a 'self-concept' questionnaire extracted from the Adjective Check

List. At the end of group sessions there was a significant mean improvement by the intervention group, compared with controls, in hospital adjustment, disease information, death perception, cancer information, group aptitude and self-concept scores. Unfortunately, less than half of the follow-up data were collected. Major limitations of this work are the apparently non-random assignment of patients to test and control groups, the use of unvalidated questionnaires and the lack of follow-up data.

A similar information-based behavioral education has been developed and assessed by Johnson (1982); it is now promoted by the American Cancer Society as a standardized course under the title 'I Can Cope'. In the Johnson study, a total of 52 patients were matched in pairs by age, sex and pretest assessment levels, then randomized into treatment and control groups; the range of diseases included was not discussed. Treatment was eight structured educational sessions each 1.5 hours long and given over four weeks by a multidisciplinary team of health professionals. Patient utilization of a 'learning resource centre' (books, tapes, filmstrips and games) was monitored. Assessment was at pre- and immediate postgroup times only, no follow-up being reported. Anxiety was measured by Spielberger's State Anxiety Inventory, meaningfulness in life by Crumbaugh's Purpose in Life Test and knowledge by a 'course enquiry' test. A statistical analysis was then made of the difference in improvement in these three scores for each matched pair (one receiving the course, the other not). Since only 22 pairs were reported, there appears to have been some attrition, which was not commented upon. Subjects in the treated group improved significantly and substantially more over the four weeks than their matched controls. This effect was not influenced by patient age or time since diagnosis. It is of interest that no significant association was found between voluntary utilization of learning resources materials and improvement scores. Weaknesses in this study include: lack of information on subject attrition and raw data scores; absence of any follow-up data; very limited assessment of mood using only an instrument designed to measure the current, probably transitory anxiety state. The improvement in knowledge of course participants, as with the study by Ferlic, Goldman and Kennedy (1979), may or may not have helped patients emotionally.

Cain *et al.* (1986) have evaluated a program which sounds very similar to Johnson's but somewhat less structured. There were eight sessions, each centered on a theme of information about cancer, ways of coping, lifestyle or communicating with others. The patients in the study were 80 women with gynecological cancer; they were assigned randomly to group intervention, individual counselling (also conducted by a social worker on the same themes and for the same time) or no counselling. Assessment was by structured interviews before, 1–2 weeks after and six months after intervention, using the Hamilton Depression and Anxiety Scales and the interview version of the Psychosocial Adjustment to Illness Scale (PAIS). Attrition was moderate and well documented. Immediately after the treatment period, those patients receiving individual attention had significantly less anxiety and depression than controls, while those in the groups had approximately the same levels as controls. By the six- month follow-up, for which data from 75 per cent of initial participants were collected, mean improvements for the individual- and group-counselled women were closely similar and significantly greater than for the untreated controls in depression, anxiety and for the total score and four of the seven subscores of the PAIS. This study is more convincing than Johnson's in its demonstration of psychosocial benefits, mainly because of the follow-up data, the use of more relevant assessment instruments and the more complete documentation of patient recruitment and drop-out. The comparison of individual with group counselling by Cain *et al.* is also valuable: while the analysis is incompletely presented, it appears that benefits were equal six months after the course but that the individual counselling produced greater effects in the shorter term.

Heinrich and Schag (1984) point to the inadequacies of the crisis/support approach to assisting many cancer patients. This dominant if usually unacknowledged treatment model assumes that patients need only be helped to reassert their normal ways of coping in response to a brief emergency, and ignores the fact that cancer often poses a series of novel and progressive problems for which many patients have insufficient coping skills. They advocate a 'behavioral medicine' approach, with evaluation of specific problems, formulation of goals, teaching new coping methods and monitoring their effectiveness. Such a program was implemented in six two-hour small group sessions (Heinrich and Schag, 1985). The sessions included evaluation, relaxation training, problem-solving and activity management techniques. A total of 51 patients with a variety of cancer types and 36 of their spouses took part in the study, participants being enrolled by groups of about 5–10 consecutive referrals into a therapy group or into a control category which received no such additional psychological care. Assignment to treatment or controls was thus non-random, although no systematic pretreatment group differences were found on subsequent analysis. Assessment of pre- and postintervention included the self-report symptom checklist of Derogatis (SCL-90-R), physician ratings of performance status on the Karnofsky scale, subjective assessment by a psychologist of what participants had done and how much benefit was experienced, together with patient ratings of quality of life (on a six-point scale), daily activities, satisfaction with current care, plus a test of knowledge about cancer. The two-month follow-up consisted only of a telephone interview enquiring about the patient's use of the techniques learned and subjective appraisal of their value.

Heinrich and Schag's results demonstrated a small, significant improvement in patients' mood between pretest and post-testing immediately after the course, as assessed by the SCL-90-R and PAIS; however, the treated group did not improve significantly more than the controls although the trends were in the expected direction. Activity also did not increase significantly, but there were treatment-related improvements in knowledge and satisfaction with care. At two-month follow-up, treated patients reported more use of coping techniques and more activity than controls. In terms of design this study suffered particularly from lack of randomization and of comprehensive follow-up data collection.

A well-designed study has recently been reported by Telch and Telch (1985, 1986). Forty-one cancer patients with mixed diagnosis who were assessed as being distressed at a preliminary interview were assigned randomly to one of three treatment conditions. The group coping skills instruction (thirteen patients, three separate small groups) consisted of six weekly 1.5 hour sessions providing instruction in relaxation, communication, problem-solving, feelings management and activity planning. The support group (fourteen patients, three groups) comprised unstructured discussions of problems, also for six sessions. The no-treatment control included fourteen patients who were, however, offered participation in 'service programmes' after the six-week period. Two therapists were used, each leading both kinds of group at different times. The authors also took the trouble to determine that patients viewed the two group modalities as equally credible, and the leaders as equally satisfactory, using a simple anonymous rating form. Assessment of the effects of the six-weeks' intervention or non-intervention was done by comparing pre- and immediate postgroup ratings using structured clinical interviews, POMS, the Cancer Inventory of Problem Situations (CIPS), an author-developed Perceived Self-Efficacy Scale and home practice records.

Telch and Telch (1986) provided detailed raw data on their results, showing a similar pre- to post-test pattern in psychological distress, perceived self-efficacy and perception of problems. The skills instruction produced large and highly significant improvements in all three scales, the support groups showed small but generally non-significant improvements, while the non-treated patients suffered significant deterioration over the six weeks. Analysis was complicated by significantly higher distress among the members of the skills training group before intervention, although an analysis of covariance assured the authors that, after adjustment for this disparity, the effects of this training were still significantly better than the other modalities. This problem in turn reflects the small numbers in the study, one of its drawbacks. It would also have been valuable to have had an intercorrelation between the outcome scores by individual patients and particularly, since the theoretical basis for the treatment was enhancement of perceived self-efficacy, a correlation of improvements in this variable with mood. The most serious limitation of this report is, however, a lack of follow-up evaluation.

(c) Conclusions on experimental studies of the psychological treatment of distress

In 1983, Watson felt that the evidence for the value of psychosocial intervention programs was 'equivocal'. Four years later it seems fair to say that the positive evidence is stronger, although, as always, more research is needed, particularly in determining what specific interventions benefit which patients. Clearly, there are methodological deficiencies in all the published work in this area; no single impeccable study exists. Major problems have been: lack of suitable control groups, of randomization or of follow-up data collection; incomplete documentation of experimental design and procedures; and the use of a variety of assessment instruments and methods, making comparison of different studies difficult (although the POMS has been quite frequently administered). The use of unvalidated or inappropriate instruments has also been common, the most insidious example of this latter practice being the testing of patients' knowledge about cancer, after an information-oriented course, without ascertaining that this new knowledge did produce useful emotional or behavioral changes.

This area of investigation appears to lag behind the best research in general psychotherapy. In part this may be a result of special difficulties in working with cancer patients; the stressors, cancer and its treatment, are usually serious and chronic, the physical and mental condition of patients is extremely variable in most experimental groups, and the disease is often progressive and fatal. Furthermore the whole concept of systematic psychological help for cancer patients (and for other people with chronic physical illness) is a relatively new one, unfamiliar as yet to many physicians and other health professionals, creating a climate in which doctors and patients are often unaware of the possible benefits of this kind of assistance. Nevertheless, stronger evidence for its efficacy has appeared in the last few years. The trend has been away from more diffuse, supportive interactions towards more structured, time-limited behavioral interventions, and recent reports are more commonly concerned with group therapy than individual work with patients. Where direct comparisons have been made, the behavioral interventions have generally been more effective than supportive therapy in alleviating psychological distress. There are insufficient data, however, to be certain that brief, behavioral, group treatment is better than longer, supportive, individual intervention, although the overwhelming economic advantages of the former favor its adoption. Individual treatment will undoubtedly continue to be needed in many situations.

(d) Studies on prolongation of life with psychological adjunctive techniques

The idea that psychological change might help in the fight against cancer has generated much publicity, and the need now seems to be for well-documented experimental trials. I am aware of five groups who have published on large series of patients receiving psychological interventions aimed explicitly at combatting the disease: these have been reviewed elsewhere (Cunningham 1984, 1986a) and will be only briefly described here.

Simonton, Mathews-Simonton and Sparks (1980) conducted a self-help education program of which a central feature was asking patients to imagine their defense systems plus medical treatment overcoming their cancer. Survival time for their patients was about twice the national (USA) median. Newton (1983) and co-workers placed more emphasis on teaching self-hypnosis, and claimed two to four times longer survival than in comparable untreated patients. Both studies are interesting and deserve consideration in my opinion, but are obviously not conclusive because the treatment groups contained highly selected individuals who may have done better than average anyway. Meares' study (1980) was also uncontrolled, describing beneficial effects, and sometimes remission, in people with advanced cancer who were taught intensive daily meditation.

A case-control trial by Morgenstern *et al.* (1984) found an improved quality of life but no significant prolongation of it in 34 women taking a self-help instruction program. A randomized control study with positive results has, however, been published by Grossarth-Maticek *et al.* (1984). They tested, in a 2×2 factorial design, the effects of both chemotherapy and 20–30 individual sessions of psychotherapy based on teaching problem-solving, examination of beliefs and expectations, relaxation and positive suggestion. The life span of randomly assigned metastatic breast cancer patients was recorded as prolonged by approximately six months on average in those receiving the psychotherapy. There was an additive effect with chemotherapy: patients receiving both treatments lived about a year longer than those getting neither.

DISCUSSION: SOME SPECULATIONS

Who needs what help, and when?

The answer to this question depends ultimately on the values and health intervention philosophies held by professionals and by the general public. According to the 'medical model', only those mentally 'sick' (i.e. obviously disturbed) should be 'treated'. There will always be a proportion of such patients requiring psychiatric care, the aim of treatment being to restore the *status quo*. On the other hand, the emerging view of behavioral medicine/ health psychology might be expressed as follows: all people with serious or life-threatening disease are under stress; many cope adequately, although their anguish may go undetected, while some manage poorly; many, perhaps almost all, can benefit from receiving adequate information, from contact with skilled and sympathetic listeners, and from educational/therapeutic approaches which allow them to cope more effectively over a long period of time with the drastic changes that cancer often brings to their lives.

Many factors will influence the introduction of such a broader program of psychosocial assistance. Perhaps the most important is cost, to be assessed against the value society puts on the emotional comfort of patients and of their families, who also often need help. Individuals may not 'want' any assistance: in some cases this stems from genuinely having adequate support and coping abilities; in others it may reflect misconceptions about the nature of psychological intervention ('that's only for crazy people') or ignorance of the possible benefits of being helped to share anxieties or to learn coping skills. In other cases, potentially valuable interventions are frustrated by the patients' need to deny to varying extents the seriousness of their condition. While this must be respected, and may be protective, it can prevent an authentic response by the patient to his condition and to the concerns of his family.

Table 2 shows stages during the progression of cancer at which various kinds of psychological help might be offered. There is already considerable evidence for the efficacy of behavioral techniques in reducing certain symptoms and side effects of cancer treatment, such as nausea and vomiting (Redd, Rosenberger and Hendler, 1983; Burish and Carey, 1984). Much more research is needed to establish the value of interventions on a wider range of quality-of-life variables, cognitive, affective, behavioral, somatic and interpersonal. Cost-effectiveness also needs to be considered, i.e. the potential for therapy to diminish subsequent requirements for health care resources.

Table 2. Main types of psychological help and when they may be useful

Type of psychosocial help	Diagnosis	First treatment	Diagnosis of recurrence	Remission	Approaching death
Crisis counselling	++	+	++	—	+
Support	++	++	++	+	++
Information	++	++	+	—	—
Existential/death counselling	—	—	+	+	++
Coping skills training					
—disability management	—	++	+	—	—
—emotional control	+	++	++	+	++
—fighting disease	+	+	++	++	—

++ often strongly needed, + possibly needed, — not usually needed. Whether or not these interventions are seen as 'needed' also depends on the patient and on the philosophy of the health care provider.

New therapeutic approaches

A standard 'behavioral package' might teach, in 4–8 sessions, communication and problem-solving skills, relaxation and activity management. Such programs have proven valuable for chronic pain (Turk, Meichenbaum and Genest, 1983) and arthritis (Lorig *et al.*, 1985) and are beginning to be explored for cancer (previous section). The manner of their presentation to patients will undoubtedly prove to be important. To this we need to add techniques that mobilize patients' deeper, more unconscious resources, e.g. self-hypnosis (Newton, 1983), meditation (Meares, 1980) and mental imagery (Simonton, Mathews-Simonton and Sparks, 1980). Imagery has received much publicity as an adjunctive therapeutic approach to cancer: whether or not it produces the imagined physiological effects, and whether or not the immune system is even important in opposing neoplastic growth, mental imagery is a potentially valuable vehicle through which patients can gain a perception of exerting some control over their disease, with benefit to their quality of life.

A variety of psychomotor and other therapies also deserve exploration, e.g. art, dance, gestalt, T'ai chi, yoga and bioenergetics. An adjunctive psychological program could offer a range of these approaches, giving patients some choice. It is important to keep an open mind on the possible usefulness of such psychological techniques, which seem at least as deserving of investigation, for their effects on quality of life, as much of the chemotherapy research on which large amounts of money are currently lavished.

Spiritual/existential issues are also of vital importance to people with cancer and other life-threatening illnesses, and should not be avoided by a mature society. Patients often need to discuss the possible meaning of their life and impending death and of the disease itself, and to attempt to gain some experience of a self-transcending order. For those who have a particular religious faith their clergy may help them with these matters; however, even non-believers may be helped spiritually by such secular techniques as life review, meditation and open-minded discussion.

A scenario for cancer care in the year 2007

The following is an intentionally provocative and idealistic sketch of a possible health care system approach to life-threatening disease at some time in the future. A theoretical rationale for such a scheme has been presented elsewhere (Cunningham, 1986b).

Since cancer is primarily a psychosocial and existential experience, the primary care person will be a 'cancer counsellor', with training in, first, clinical psychological techniques, secondly, existential matters, and thirdly with some knowledge of the basic biology and medical treatment of cancer. He or she might have had primary training in medicine, nursing, psychology, theology, social work or other areas, with appropriate postgraduate work. The cancer counsellor will be responsible for overall coordination of care and for continuing support and advice to the patient. Appropriate rumuneration will reward this demanding role! Medical specialists will of course be responsible for physical diagnosis and treatment of the patient, but as consultants rather than primary care providers. Alleviation of emotional distress in the patient and his or her family will receive as much attention as the relief of physical pain. Psychiatric and spiritual consultants (e.g. clergy) will be called in as needed. The patient will be encouraged to face the situation honestly and to take an active part in coping and disease-fighting. To this end he or she will, along with a mutually supportive peer group, be offered a wide variety of self-help strategies in a gentle, non-victimizing manner that will foster a sense of dignity and personal psychological mastery over adversity.

SUMMARY

There is an increasing tendency to offer systematic psychosocial care to alleviate emotional distress in cancer patients. A trend is beginning to be discernible, away from earlier relative neglect, towards supportive interventions, to teaching active skills for emotional coping, and even perhaps towards teaching ways of fighting the disease psychologically. The experimental literature on relief of dysphoric mood through individual and group interventions has been reviewed: it is concluded that although, as always, more research is needed, the evidence supports the view derived from clinical experience and commonsense that such interventions may help many patients.

REFERENCES

Bloom, J. R., Ross, R. D., and Burnell, G. (1978). The effect of social support on patient adjustment after breast surgery, *Patient Counselling Health Education*, **1**, 50–59.

Buchanan, D. (1978). Group therapy for chronic physically ill patients, *Psychosomatics*, **19**, 425–431.

Burish, T. G., and Carey, M. P. (1984). Conditioned responses to cancer chemotherapy: etiology and treatment, in *Impact of Psychoendocrine Systems in Cancer and Immunity* (Eds B. H. Fox and B. H. Newberry), C. J. Hogrefe, New York, pp. 147–178.

Cain, E. N., Kohorn, E. I., Quinlan, D. M., Latimer, K., and Schwartz, P. E. (1986). Psychosocial benefits of a cancer support group, *Cancer*, **57**, 183–189.

Capone, M. A., Westie, K. S., Chitwood, J. S., Feigenbaum, D., and Good, R. S.

(1979). Crisis intervention: a functional model for hospitalized cancer patients, *Am. J. Orthopsychiat.*, **49**, 598–607.

Cunningham, A. J. (1984). Psychotherapy for cancer: a review, *Advances*, **1**, 8–14.

Cunningham, A. J. (1985). The influence of mind on cancer, *Can. Psychol.*, **26**, 13–29.

Cunningham, A. J. (1986a). Psychological self-help by cancer patients, in *Coping with Cancer Stress* (Ed. B. A. Stoll), Martinus Nijhoff, The Netherlands, pp. 131–142.

Cunningham, A. J. (1986b). Information and health in the many levels of man. Towards a more comprehensive theory of health and disease, *Advances*, **3**, 32–45.

Derogatis, L. R., Morrow, G. R., Fetting, J., Penman, D., Piasetsky, S., Schmale, A. M., Henrichs, M., and Carnicke, C. L. M. (1983). The prevalence of psychiatric disorders among cancer patients, *J. Am. Med. Assoc.*, **249**, 751–759.

Farash, J. L. (1979). Effect of counselling on resolution of loss and body image disturbance following a mastectomy, *Dissertation Abstracts International*, **39B**, 4027.

Ferlic, M., Goldman, A., and Kennedy, B. J. (1979). Group counselling in adult patients with advanced cancer, *Cancer*, **43**, 760–766.

Forester, B., Kornfeld, D. S., and Fleiss, J. L. (1985). Psychotherapy during radiotherapy: effects on emotional and physical distress, *Am. J. Psychiat.*, **142**, 22–27.

Friedenbergs, I., Gordon, W., Hibbard, M., Levine, L., Wolf, C., and Diller, L. (1981–82). Psychosocial aspects of living with cancer: a review of the literature, *Int. J. Psychiat. Med.*, **11**, 303–329.

Golonka, L. M. (1977). The use of group counselling with breast cancer patients receiving chemotherapy, *Dissertation Abstracts International*, **37** (10-A), 6362.

Gordon, M. W., Freidenbergs, I., Diller, L., Hibbard, M., Wolf, C., Levine, L., Lipkins, R., Ezrachi, O., and Lucido, D. (1980). Efficacy of psychosocial intervention with cancer patients, *J. Consult. Clin. Psychol.*, **48**, 743–759.

Greer, S., and Silberfarb, P. M. (1982). Psychological concomitants of cancer: current state of research, *Psychol. Med.*, **12**, 563–573.

Grossarth-Maticek, R., Schmidt, P., Vetter, H., and Arndt, S. (1984). Psychotherapy research in oncology, in *Health Care and Human Behaviour* (Eds A. Steptoe and A. Mathews), Academic Press, New York, pp. 325–341.

Heinrich, R. L., and Schag, C. C. (1984). A behavioral medicine approach to coping with cancer: a case report, *Cancer Nursing*, June, 243–247.

Heinrich, R. L., and Schag, C. C. (1985). Stress and activity management: group treatment for cancer patients and spouses, *J. Consult. Clin. Psychol.*, **53**, 439–446.

Holland, J. C., and Rowland, J. H. (1981). Psychiatric, psychosocial and behavioral interventions in the treatment of cancer, in *Perspectives on Behavioural Medicine* (Ed. S. M. Weiss), Academic Press, New York, pp. 235–260.

Jacobs, C., Ross, R. D., Walker, I. M., and Stockdale, F. W. (1983). Behavior of cancer patients: a randomized study of the effects of education and peer support groups, *Am. J. Clin. Oncol.*, **6**, 347–353.

Johnson, J. (1982). The effects of a patient education course on persons with a chronic illness, *Cancer Nursing*, April, 117–123.

Koenig, R., Levine, S. M., and Brenna, M. J. (1967). The emotional status of cancer patients as measured by a psychological test, *J. Chronic Dis.*, **20**, 923–930.

Linn, M. W., Linn, B. S., and Harris, R. (1982). Effects of counselling for late stage cancer patients, *Cancer*, **49**, 1048–1055.

Lorig, K., Lubeck, D., Kraines, R. G., Seleznick, M., and Holman, H. R. (1985). Outcomes of self-help education for patients with arthritis, *Arthritis Rheumatism*, **28**, 680–5.

Maguire, P., Tait, A., Brooke, M., Thomas, C., and Sellwood, R. (1980). Effect of counselling on the psychiatric morbidity associated with mastectomy, *Brit. Med. J.*, **281**, 1455–1460.

Meares, A. (1980). What can the cancer patient expect from intensive meditation? *Austral. Fam. Physician*, **9**, 322–325.

Meyerowitz, B. E. (1980). Psychosocial correlates of breast cancer and its treatment, *Psychol. Bull.*, **87**, 108–131.

Morgenstern, H., Gellert, G. A., Walter, S. D., Ostgeld, A. M., and Siegel, B. S. (1984). The impact of a psychosocial support program on survival with breast cancer: the importance of selection bias in program eveluation, *J. Chronic Dis.*, **37**, 273–82.

Newton, B. W. (1982–3). The use of hypnosis in the treatment of cancer patients, *Am. J. Clin. Hypnosis*, **25**, 104–113.

Novack, D. H., Plumer, R., Smith, R. L., Ochitill, H., Morrow, G. R., and Bennett, J. M. (1979). Changes in physicians' attitudes towards telling the cancer patient, *J. Am. Med. Assoc.*, **241**, 897–900.

Petty, F., and Noyes, R. (1981). Depression secondary to cancer, *Biol. Psychiat.*, **16**, 1203–1209.

Redd, W. H., Rosenberger, P. H., and Hendler, C. S. (1983). Controlling chemotherapy side effects, *Am. J. Clin. Hypnosis*, **25**, 161–72.

Ringler, K., Whitman, H., Gustafson, J., and Coleman, F. (1981). Technical advances in leading a cancer patient group, *Int. J. Group Psychother.*, **31**, 329–343.

Schipper, H., Clinch, J., McMurray, A., and Levitt, M. (1984). Measuring the quality of life of cancer patients: the Functional Living Index—Cancer: development and validation, *J. Clin. Oncol.*, **2**, 472–483.

Schwartz, M. D. (1977). An information and discussion program for women after a mastectomy, *Arch. Gen. Surg.*, **112**, 276–281.

Simonton, O. C., Mathews-Simonton, S., and Sparks, T. F. (1980). Psychological intervention in the treatment of cancer, *Psychosomatics*, **21**, 226–233.

Spiegel, D., Bloom, J. R., and Yalom, I. (1981). Group support for patients with metastatic cancer, *Arch. Gen. Psychiat.*, **38**, 527–533.

Spiegel, D., and Yalom, I. D. (1978). A support group for dying patients, *Int. J. Group Psychother.*, **28**, 233–245.

Tarrier, N., and Maguire, P. (1984). Treatment of psychological distress following mastectomy: an initial report, *Behav. Res. Therapy*, **22**, 81–84.

Telch, C. F., and Telch, M. J. (1985). Psychological approaches for enhancing coping among cancer patients: a review, *Clin. Psychol. Rev.*, **5**, 325–344.

Telch, C. F., and Telch, M. J. (1986). Group coping skills instruction and supportive group therapy for cancer patients: a comparison of strategies, *J. Consult. Clin. Psychol.*, **54**, 802–808.

Temoshok, L., and Heller, B. W. (1984). On comparing apples, oranges and fruit salad: a methodological overview of medical outcome studies in psychosocial oncology, in *Psychosocial Stress and Cancer* (Ed. C. L. Cooper), John Wiley & Sons, Chichester, pp. 231–260.

Turk, D. C., Meichenbaum, D., and Genest, M. (1983). *Pain and Behavioral Medicine*, Guildford Press, London.

Vachon, M. L. S., Lyall, W. A. L., Rogers, J., Cochrane, J., and Freeman, S. J. (1981–2). The effectiveness of psychosocial support during post-surgical treatment of breast cancer, *Int. J. Psychiat. Med.*, **11**, 365–372.

Ware, J. E. (1984). Conceptualizing disease impact and treatment outcomes, *Cancer*, **53**, 2316–2323.

Watson, M. (1983). Psychosocial intervention with cancer patients: a review, *Psychol. Med.*, **13**, 839–46.

Weisman, A. D., and Worden, J. W. (1976). The existential plight in cancer: significance of the first 100 days, *Int. J. Psychiat. Med.*, **7**, 1–12.

Weisman, A. D., and Worden, J. W. (1977). Coping and Vulnerability in Cancer Patients, Research report, funded by National Cancer Institute, USA.

Weisman, A. D., Worden, J. W., and Sobel, H. J. (1980). Psychosocial Screening and Intervention with Cancer Patients, Research report, Boston, privately printed.

West, B. L. (1981). Cognitive–behavioral analysis system of psychotherapy (C-BASP) as applied to depression in a cancer population, *Dissertation Abstracts International*, **41**, 3595B.

Wood, P. E., Milligan, M., Christ, D., and Liff, D. (1978). Group counselling for cancer patients in a community hospital, *Psychosomatics*, **19**, 555–561.

Worden, J. W. (1983). Psychosocial screening of cancer patients, *J. Psychosoc. Oncol.*, **1**, 1–10.

Worden, J. W., and Weisman, A. D. (1980). Do cancer patients really want counselling? *Gen. Hosp. Psychiat.*, **2**, 2–15.

Worden, J. W., and Weisman, A. D. (1984). Preventive psychosocial intervention with newly diagnosed cancer patients, *Gen. Hosp. Psychiat.*, **6**, 243–249.

Yalom, I. D., and Greaves, C. (1977). Group therapy with the terminally ill, *Am. J. Psychiat.*, **134**, 396–400.

Youssef, F. A. (1984). Crisis intervention: a group therapy approach for hospitalized breast cancer patients, *J. Advanced Nursing*, **9**, 307–313.

Stress and Breast Cancer
Edited by C. L. Cooper
© 1988 John Wiley & Sons Ltd

Chapter 8
Breast Cancer—A Family Affair

Lea A. Baider
Department of Clinical Oncology and Radiotherapy, Hadassah University Hospital, Jerusalem, Israel
and
Atara Kaplan De-Nour
Department of Psychiatry, Hadassah University Hospital, Jerusalem, Israel

Events in the life of an individual need to be understood in terms of time and space, where time refers to personal developmental phases and space to the person's sociocultural environment, his 'microsociety'. The smallest context of the person's own self and his social identity relates to his family and, for the purpose of this study, to the marital couple.

The subject of this exploratory study is couple interaction and adjustment to a life-threatening event, the event being the detection of cancer, specifically breast cancer, followed by either lumpectomy or mastectomy.

In the forefront of research on the psychological effect of cancer, Holland (1976), Bard and Sutherland (1977) and Holland and Mastrovito (1980) outlined a spectrum of factors that contribute to 'good' or 'poor' adjustment in breast cancer patients. According to their findings the sociocultural and interpersonal environment of the patient is particularly important in the process of adaptation. The response of a partner to a woman after breast cancer and mastectomy can either provide her with, or deprive her of, the security of being loved and esteemed despite the presence of significant illness.

Holland and Jacobs (1986) referred to three key issues in the psychological adaptation of women to breast cancer. First, variables in the life stage in which the event occurs; second, the woman's previous emotional stability, her personality and coping style; and third, the presence and availability of interpersonal support. Recognizing the importance of each one of these factors, for the purpose of the present study we will concentrate only on interpersonal support, specifically husband–wife interaction.

The woman's perception of her husband's role in the marriage, fluctuating from very positive to very critical, can be fundamental for her self-esteem; he may be viewed as either providing or denying support. The husband's support and empathy play a large part in the emotional recovery of his partner. The interplay of the presence or absence of social support in a patient's environment appears to be as important an influence for the main-tenance of psychological comfort as the woman's own intrapsychic resources (Bloom, 1982a; Revenson, Wollman and Felton, 1983; Goldberg and Wool, 1985).

Being married has been shown to be a good predictor of adjustment to health problems in general, and specifically to adjustment following mastec-tomy (Bard, 1952; Grandstaff, 1976; Jamison, Wellisch and Pasnau, 1978; Lindsey *et al.*, 1981). However, contrary to most clinical and epidemiological studies, Bloom (1982a) did not find marital status to be a significant predictor of adjustment, contending that it is the perception of support rather than the existence of formal social ties which is critical. Maguire's (1975) findings would seem to support this view. A critical or unsympathetic response from the husband could result in a psychological mechanism of avoidance behavior and social isolation on the part of the patient. In contrast, husbands who reaffirmed their love and who refused to allow either concealment of the scar, social withdrawal or avoidance of sexual contact, supported the morale of their partners and helped them to recover.

The expectation of breast cancer patients, and indeed of the helping professions, that the marital partner will and should be a source of support may not, however, be realistic, particularly if the quality of the relationship before mastectomy was unstable, ambivalent and conflictual. While Wabrek and Wabrek (1976) stated that even a good marriage cannot easily survive the trauma of mastectomy, Maguire (1975) found that the great strain that was placed on the marriage resulted in the couple being brought closer together.

Lichtman, Wood and Taylor (1982) found that the marital relationship of breast cancer patients was significantly affected by the quality of the relation-ship prior to diagnosis. Other influencing factors were the quality of the couple's current sexual relationship, type of cancer surgery, the husband's own reaction to the cancer, and the degree of honest and open communi-cation between the partners.

It may be suggested, therefore, that the husband's reaction and adjustment are often critically important to the breast cancer patient (Joiner and Fisher, 1981; Funch and Mettlin, 1982). In one of the first studies on this subject, Jamison, Wellisch and Pasnau (1978) administered a questionnaire to 41 postmastectomy women, finding that 23 per cent had not allowed themselves to be seen naked by their spouses following operation, 14.3 per cent had not had intercourse with their spouses and an additional 24 per cent of the women reported that they had less sexual satisfaction in their relationship since mastectomy. Wellish, Jamison and Pasnau (1978) did a comparison study, using the same instruments as Jamison *et al.* (1978), for a group of men whose wives or partners had had a mastectomy. Only 31 of these men responded to a mailed questionnaire—a response rate of only 15 per cent: 57 per cent of the men reported involvement in presurgical decisions while 43 per cent reported very little or no involvement; 73 per cent were satisfied with the amount of involvement but 23 per cent would have liked more involvement. Furthermore, a significant number of men reported psychosomatic and psychological reactions, e.g. sleep disorders, loss of appetite and work disruption during the time of diagnosis and treatment.

In a more recent study (not very conclusive due to the small and self-selective sample), Plummer (1985) investigated the changes that occur in the intimate relationship of couples after the female partner has undergone mastectomy. Ten mastectomy patients and their partners, and two control groups, were interviewed before and two months after surgery. The results showed that male partners of mastectomy patients become less satisfied with sexual adjustment postsurgically and more dissatisfied with aspects of couples' affective communication.

Similar findings were presented by Johnstone-Wyatt (1981), who conducted a survey on 83 mastectomy couples and on a comparison group of non-surgical couples. The data confirmed the hypothesis that mastectomy couples would report more sexual concerns and needs, have poorer global sexual adjustment and would express more frequently a need for help than comparison couples. They also confirmed the assumption that partners of mastectomy women would express more frequently a need to learn how to be caring and loving when their partners are ill than comparison males.

The basic recurring theme of 'why me' of women with breast cancer has been extensively considered in many studies, but surprisingly limited research has been performed concerning the same question in relation to the partner and the couple. From the husband's point of view we believe that there exists more than just a semantic differentiation: 'Why is this happening to her?' 'Why is this happening to me?' and 'Why is this happening to us?' We can only presume that this is perhaps a sociocultural pattern in terms of the role men play in society rather than just a psychological reaction to the situation (Sabo, Brown and Smith, 1986). Men are usually perceived by society as caretakers, copers, as taking care of the wife in the specific roles of instrumental tasks. It may be normative assumptions, cultural or more habitual to think within this pattern of social behavior, making a clear division between the victim and the rescuer, the weak and the strong, the instrumental and the emotional tasks.

Goldberg *et al.* (1984), however, provide a counterbalance by assuming that it is sometimes overlooked that the experience of breast cancer creates tremendous stress not only for the patient but also for the spouse, who frequently will have to assume the role of supporter. Thus the husband may have great difficulties in providing support to a partner with a life-threatening disease, particularly if his own need for support is unmet.

One can say that there is general agreement that family, and especially partner, support is a major factor in the adjustment of women with breast cancer. Moreover, there seems in addition to be agreement that breast cancer is also stressful for the husband. It is surprising, therefore, that so few studies focus on the dyadic relationship, considering breast cancer patients and spouses simultaneously. In an earlier study Baider and Kaplan De-Nour (1984) reported on 20 postmastectomy women and their husbands who were examined for adjustment and family relations. It was found that the husbands had nearly as many adjustment problems as the women. Furthermore, a strong relationship was found between the adjustment of the women and their husbands.

SUBJECTS AND METHODS

Thirty-five postlumpectomy and 27 postmastectomy women and their husbands formed the present study group. The postlumpectomy group included all the married women who were in follow-up at the Oncological Institute of the Hadassah University Hospital in Jerusalem. These women were not in active treatment and had no signs of active disease, and their husbands agreed to participate in a study on adjustment to breast cancer. The postmastectomy women were selected by the same criteria from a much larger pool. The two groups were similar in terms of background, age and education, and a similar time had elapsed since surgery. Table 1 presents the medical information about the 62 patients.

Table 1. Medical information

Treatment	$T_1 N_0$	$T_2 N_0$	$T_1 N_1/T_2 N_1$	Total
A Lumpectomy + radiation	13	13	1	27
B Lumpectomy + radiation + chemotherapy	2	2	6	10
C Mastectomy	3	7	0	10
D Mastectomy + chemotherapy	2	6	7	15
Total	20	28	14	62

A previous study (Baider, Rizel and Kaplan De-Nour, 1986) showed that there are no substantial differences in adjustment between postlumpectomy and postmastectomy women once age, education and time since operation are controlled. In the present study, therefore, the postlumpectomy and the postmastectomy couples were handled as one group.

The time since breast surgery was a mean of one and a half years (with a standard deviation of 14.7 months). Table 2 presents the couples' background.

Table 2. Breast cancer couples—background

	Patients		Husbands		Pearson	p	T value	p
	x	SD	x	SD				
Age	46.9	9.47	50.8	10.14	0.923	0.000	−7.74	0.000
Education	13.7	3.09	14.6	3.20	0.341	0.008	−1.89	0.063

The couples were contacted by telephone and subsequently interviewed in their homes by a research assistant. After receiving their agreement to participate in a study on adjustment to breast cancer, the two partners were presented with identical batches of five self-reports which they answered separately.

Two measures were used to assess psychological condition: the Beck Depression Inventory (BDI) (Beck and Beamesderfer, 1974) and the Spielberger Trait State Anxiety Scale (STAS) (Spielberger, Gorsuch and Lushen, 1970). Derogatis' Psychosocial Adjustment to Illness Scale (PAIS) (Derogatis and Lopez, 1983) was used to measure impact of disease. This questionnaire is composed of items that cover the domains of adjustment, i.e. health care orientation, vocational environment, domestic environment, sexual relations, extended family relations, social environment and psychological distress. It provides information about global adjustment as well as about these seven specific areas. In some of the sections the items are phrased 'your illness', etc. In the husband's self-report these sentences were rephrased to 'your wife's illness', thus taping the impact of the wife's illness on the husband's functioning or feelings.

In these three self-reports—BDI, STAS and PAIS—higher scores indicate more problems.

Two measures were used to assess resource variables. The Shanan Sentence Completion Technique (SSCT) (Shanan, 1973; Shanan, Kaplan De-Nour and Garty, 1976) was used to assess coping. This is a semiprojective test composed of 40 stem sentences that have to be completed. The 40 items cover four categories (each of ten items). Category I assesses a person's goals and aims, Category II sources of difficulties and frustration, Category III a person's tendency to cope actively or passively with taxing situations, and Category IV self-image. In addition to the four specific facets of coping, the test provides information about the person's total coping capabilities, higher scores indicating better coping. The test is also scored for directions of investment of cachectic energy into interpersonal relations (P), instrumental activities (O) or narcissistically in the self (-S). Furthermore the test provides a measure for defensiveness and/or lack of cooperation (R) represented by vague, uncommitted completions or straight rejections (not completing the stem sentence). Since the test is semiprojective, it usually creates more resistance and some subjects refuse to answer it.

The last self-report is Moos' Family Environment Scale (FES) (Moos and Moos, 1981), which provides information about the person's perception of his family environment. This self-report is composed of 90 items, answered by true/false, which are grouped into ten scales. The perception of the relationship is taped by three scales—Cohesion, Expressiveness and Conflict. The personal growth aspect is taped by five scales, i.e. Independence, Achievement Orientation, Cultural–Intellectual Orientation, Active Recreational Orientation and Moral–Religious Orientation. The system is represented by two scales, i.e. Organization and Control.

In order to be able to look for similarities/differences between partners, all data were analyzed by paired *t*-test between patients and husbands as well as by Pearson correlations.

RESULTS

Table 3 presents the couples' psychological condition. The women were found to be significantly more depressed than their husbands. Significant correlations were found between partners both in depression and in anxiety.

Table 3. Psychological condition

	Patients		Husbands		Pearson	p	T value	p
	x	SD	x	SD				
Anxiety T	40.8	10.46	39.2	11.50	0.144	NS	0.55	NS
Anxiety S	39.9	8.01	37.2	9.65	0.273	0.033	1.89	0.063
Depression	6.8	5.92	4.2	4.51	0.391	0.003	3.36	0.001

Table 4 presents the adjustment of the couples as assessed along the PAIS. On most domains of adjustment the husbands reported somewhat more problems, and in the section of health care orientation the difference was of statistical significance. Very strong positive correlations between partners were found in the domains of domestic environment, sexual relations and extended family relations, indicating that both were inclined to report similar levels of problems.

Table 4. Psychosocial adjustment

PAIS domain	N	Patients (women)		Husbands		Pearson		T value	2-tail prob.
		x	SD	x	SD	Corr.	Prob.		
I Health care	62	5.5	2.76	6.9	3.51	0.035	NS	−2.66	0.010
II Vocational environment	55	1.7	1.89	2.3	2.04	0.232	0.089	−1.71	0.092
III Domestic environment	60	2.7	2.51	2.5	2.51	0.551	0.000	0.57	NS
IV Sexual relations	61	1.8	2.60	1.9	2.47	0.602	0.000	−0.12	NS
V Extended family	62	0.5	1.25	0.6	1.02	0.495	0.000	−0.44	NS
VI Social environment	61	1.0	2.51	1.6	2.36	0.148	NS	−1.45	0.152
VII Psychological distress	59	4.3	3.15	3.5	2.67	0.055	NS	1.43	0.159
Total		17.1	10.95	19.1	10.49	0.358	0.004	−1.30	0.200

The results of the groups' coping are presented in Table 5. The husbands were somewhat more defensive (higher score on R) but they manifested significantly better coping. The husbands also invested significantly less energy in the self.

Table 5. Coping (43 breast cancer couples)

SSCT category	Patients (women)		Husbands		T value	2-tail prob.
	x	SD	x	SD		
I Goal and aims	5.2	1.92	5.5	1.90	−0.94	0.350
II Sources of difficulty	3.6	1.54	4.1	1.73	−1.40	0.170
III Active coping	3.5	2.09	4.8	2.40	−3.32	0.002
IV Self-image	5.3	1.92	5.8	1.78	−1.17	0.248
Total	17.8	5.01	21.8	7.15	−3.48	0.001
Investment of energy into						
P Interpersonal relations	5.2	2.31	5.7	2.16	−1.23	0.227
O Instrumental activities	3.5	2.40	3.9	2.37	−0.88	0.382
S Self	6.3	2.04	4.2	2.45	5.12	0.000
R Rejection	5.0	4.12	6.9	5.86	−1.75	0.087

The results on the Family Environment Scale are presented in Figure 1. The perception of the family of both wives and husbands falls well within the range of normal (American norms) families. No significant differences were found between the women and husbands. The women reported somewhat less organization and expressiveness and somewhat more active recreation, cultural orientation, independence and conflict. Only on three of the ten scales were the correlations between the partners not statistically significant.

We looked into factors that could influence adjustment. As to background,

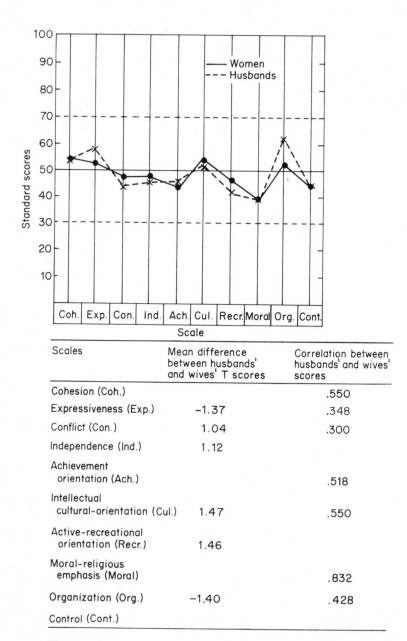

Scales	Mean difference between husbands' and wives' T scores	Correlation between husbands' and wives' scores
Cohesion (Coh.)		.550
Expressiveness (Exp.)	−1.37	.348
Conflict (Con.)	1.04	.300
Independence (Ind.)	1.12	
Achievement orientation (Ach.)		.518
Intellectual cultural-orientation (Cul.)	1.47	.550
Active-recreational orientation (Recr.)	1.46	
Moral-religious emphasis (Moral)		.832
Organization (Org.)	−1.40	.428
Control (Cont.)		

Figure 1: Social climate scale profile. Family Environment Scale.

in the women's group age had practically no influence on adjustment (only positive correlations of 0.263, $p = 0.041$ with problems in sexual relations) nor did education (only negative correlation—0.268 with depression). No relationship at all was found between the time since operation and the adjustment measures. In the husbands' group neither age nor education had any influence on adjustment. Time since operation also had no influence.

Coping as assessed by the SSCT had no influence on anxiety and depression in either group (patients and husbands).

The influence of coping on adjustment as reported along the PAIS was minimal. In the women's group only a few significant correlations were found: problems in health care orientation were correlated with self-image (−0.370), problems in vocational environment were related to active coping (−0.323) and to investment of energy in interpersonal relations (−0.370), and problems in the social environment were correlated with investment of energy in interpersonal relations (−0.309).

In the husbands' group the relationship between coping and adjustment was stronger. A significant relationship was found between active coping and the total PAIS score (−0.314), the strongest relationship being with problems in the domestic environment (−0.318). Self-image was found to be related to problems in the social environment (−0.393).

We looked into the relationship of adjustment and perception of the family. On the whole not many significant relationships were found between the FES subscales and anxiety and depression. State anxiety was significantly correlated with cohesion (−0.274 in the patients' group and −0.320 in the husbands' group). In the husbands' group a significant correlation was found also between state anxiety and moral–religious orientation (−0.308) as well as with organization (−0.280). In the women's group a significant correlation was found between state anxiety and control (−0.280). The significant relationships of depression and perception of family environment were minimal: in the patients' group only with expressiveness (−0.371) and in the husbands' group with cohesion (−0.381) and with achievement orientation (−0.350). Much stronger relationships were found between adjustment (as reported on the PAIS) and family environment, especially the relationship scales (Table 6). Only the significant, or near significant (in brackets) correlations were included in the table. One can see that the two domains of adjustment most linked to perception of family environment are those of sexual relations (both in patients' and husbands' groups) and domestic environment (especially in the husbands' group). Furthermore it should be noted that there was quite a strong negative correlation between the incongruence score, i.e. the difference between the partners' perception of their family and the husbands' adjustment, as opposed to the women's adjustment.

Table 6. Adjustment and family relations

	Cohesion		Expressiveness		Conflict		Incongruence score	
PAIS domain	Pts	Husbands	Pts	Husbands	Pts	Husbands	Pts	Husbands
I Health care orientation	−0.302							
III Domestic environment	−0.402	−0.299		−0.276		0.295		(0.256)
IV Sexual relations	−0.279	−0.315	−0.278	−0.261	0.296	0.266	0.278	
VI Social environment	−0.296							(0.244)
VIII Psychological distress		−0.296	−0.291					0.283
Total PAIS	−0.403	(−0.240)	−0.283	−0.290				0.270

In order to reach some understanding about the influence of the medical condition on adjustment, we compared the patients diagnosed Stage I to those diagnosed Stage II. The two groups did not differ in background, coping and family relations. On the adjustment measures no differences were found between the Stage I and Stage II patients (except for a tendency of more problems in the social environment in the Stage II group, 2.1 compared with 0.7, $t = 1.26$, $p = 0.227$).

The husbands of the Stage II women were somewhat less satisfied with the medical treatment (on health care orientation 8.4 compared with 6.5, $t = 1.68$, $p = 0.109$). No differences were found in coping and in adjustment between the husbands of Stage I women and those of Stage II. The latter, however, described a different family environment, with more cohesion ($\times$ 7.9 compared with 6.9, $t = 2.16$, $p = 0.040$), more independence ($\times$ 6.9 compared with 5.8, $t = 2.72$, $p = 0.014$) and a tendency for more orientation ($\times$ 6.9 compared with 6.4, $t = 1.51$, $p = 0.143$) and more control ($\times$ 4.5 compared with 3.3, $t = 1.40$, $p = 0.187$).

We compared the patients who had also undergone chemotherapy with those who had not. The two groups did not differ in terms of age, education or time since surgery, nor in any of the adjustment measures; the only tendency to a difference was that the patients who had had chemotherapy were somewhat less depressed (5.5 compared to 7.81, $t = -1.53$, $p = 0.131$). No significant differences were found in coping and in perception of the family environment. We did find differences between the husbands of the women who had had chemotherapy and the husbands of those who had not had chemotherapy. The postchemotherapy husbands had significantly fewer problems in the extended family relation ($\times$ 0.1 compared with 0.9, $t = 3.80$,

$p = 0.000$) and fewer problems in the social environment ($\times$ 0.8 compared with 2.2, $t = -2.12$, $p = 0.009$). These husbands were also significantly less anxious (state anxiety $\times$ 34.0 compared with 40.0, $t = -2.60$, $p = 0.012$). Few differences were found in coping: the postchemotherapy husbands were lower in 'goals and aims) (4.7 compared with 5.8, $t = -2.07$, $p = 0.044$), and the same tendency was found on the total score (19.4 compared with 22.5, $t = -1.56$, $p = 0.127$). No statistically significant differences were found in the perception of the family in the two groups.

Thus it seems that stage of disease as well as history of chemotherapy had no influence on the women's adjustment. On the other hand, these factors seem to be connected to the husbands' adjustment.

DISCUSSION

We studied 62 couples where the wife was ill with breast cancer, investigating the psychological condition, psychosocial adjustment, coping and family relations of both partners.

On the whole the group was fairly well adjusted. Only nine of the 62 women (14.5 per cent) and eight of the husbands reported what could be regarded as clinical depression. Meyerowitz (1980) stated that the most common psychological reaction to breast cancer is depression, but the incidence and severity of depression reported varies considerably. The literature on the psychological aspects of breast cancer estimates that as many as 24–30 per cent of women undergoing mastectomy will have psychological problems sufficiently serious to require psychiatric evaluation (Bloom, 1982b; Hughes, 1982). Jamison, Wellisch and Pasnau (1978) found depression to be a considerable problem in postmastectomy women. Almost 25 per cent of the women stated that they had suicidal ideation after surgery and 14.6 per cent reported having sought professional help for psychological problems related to breast cancer. Silberfarb, Maurer and Crouthamel (1980), on the other hand, disputed previous findings and reported that in their study postmastectomy women did not suffer from depression. They distinguished between 'depressive illness', which they did not find in postmastectomy women, and 'depressive affect', which was noted in 15 per cent of their patients. Patients' and husbands' scores on anxiety were also around T score of 50 (Israeli norms).

In the present study patients' and husbands' adjustment problems as reported along the PAIS were moderate (T score of 50 when using Derogatis' norms for mixed cancers). Patients' and husbands' coping was also fairly high, much higher than found, for example, in dialysis patients (Shanan, Kaplan De-Nour and Garty, 1976).

Thus it seems that both patients and husbands were indeed well adjusted, i.e. non-depressed, non-anxious and with not too many adjustment problems.

These results inevitably raise the question of why such good adjustment was found. There are a few possible explanations. First of all there is the question of credibility: to what extent did patients and husbands fully report their difficulties? We are inclined to believe that they did not hold back or suppress information: they addressed the task seriously, hardly any item was not answered, and they seemed involved in the self-reports.

It might well be that this good adjustment was found because we studied the best patients at their best time; we studied a group with reasonably high education, married and with moderately good marital conditions. Family relations came out as normal, and communication between husband and wife was free enough to allow for both partners to participate in the study. Women who did not allow us to interview their husbands or whose husbands refused to participate were not included in the present report. In addition, at the time of the study none of the women were in active treatment nor did they show any signs of active disease. One could conclude and suggest, therefore, that at least during remission, the couples' adjustment is quite good and they return to routine life.

Yet, in both groups of patients and husbands, a rather high variability was found, with some people doing extremely well and some extremely poorly.

From the information available to us we tried to gain some further understanding of this variability in adjustment. Background in terms of age and education had practically no influence on adjustment. A somewhat surprising finding was that medical history in terms of time since operation, stage of cancer and chemotherapy had no effect at all on the women's adjustment (Knobf, 1986; Meyerowitz, 1980). However, surprisingly, the medical history seems to have influenced the husbands' adjustment. It seems as if the post-chemotherapy husbands feel more secure and have fewer adjustment problems than the husbands of women who did not have chemotherapy.

In previous studies of medically ill patients, a strong relationship was found between coping and adjustment measures (Mechanic, 1974; Miller, 1983; Corbin and Strauss, 1984). In studies of healthy populations in stress, a very strong relationship was found between adjustment and coping (Steinglass, Kaplan De-Nour and Shye, 1985). Therefore we were quite surprised that only marginal relationships were found in the present study, minimal in the patients and more substantial in their husbands. A possible explanation for this limited influence of coping on adjustment lies in the finding that another factor, i.e. family relations, had a stronger and perhaps overwhelming influence. Perception of the family environment, especially perceived cohesion, was found to correlate strongly with the adjustment measures used. Furthermore, strong intracouple agreement about the level of adjustment problems was found. Thus it could be that in the group studied (selected on the basis of couples agreeing to participate in a psychological study of breast cancer), family relations and one partner adjustment have a stronger impact on the second partner adjustment than his/her own coping capabilities.

Another major finding was that on every measure of adjustment but self-report of depression, the husbands reported as many problems as the women with breast cancer. This finding, together with the previous one, raises the question of cause and effect. Which of the partners is the first to show adjustment problems and who is the reactor? This question is of crucial importance if we wish to plan effective interventions. Should one treat the patients or the husbands or is it different in different couples, i.e. in one couple the wife is the initiator of stress and in another couple the husband is the cause of difficulties. Our study, by design, cannot provide an answer to this question. It emphasizes, however, what was suggested by Goldberg and Wool (1985), that the husband, being in a stressful situation, might not be able to supply the support needed by the couple. Actually it also confirms what was expressed by Weisman and Worden (1977), that, as cancer spreads throughout the body, it also spreads into social and emotional domains, challenging life's values and disrupting families. Since the family is both a part of the patient's environment and a potential source of social support, patient and family are intricately enmeshed in the coping process (Chekryn, 1984; Gotay, 1984).

A major theme in the literature of breast cancer is that the ill person does not progress through the experience of the illness alone, but that the patient is part of a dyadic system where members mutually affect one another.

Throughout the last two decades the literature on breast cancer focused on just one side of the picture—the difficulties of women in coping with illness, the emotional handicaps which illness produces, better or worse coping mechanisms of the patients and its profound meaning in terms of better adaptation and quality of life (Taylor, Lichtman and Wood, 1984; Metzger, Rogers and Bauman, 1983; Gottschalk and Hoigard-Martin, 1986; Holland and Jacobs, 1986).

The medical definition of the patient is as of a single organism: the individual with the physical signs and symptoms of disease. One can assume that most patients live in some kind of family system, and that a vast majority of breast cancer patients have a partner. It is perhaps paradoxical, therefore, that a process of disassociation of the patient from the partner is maintained.

We may have widened our vision sufficiently to be able to look at interpersonal as well as intrapsychic factors affecting the patient, but we generally fail to see them as an active part of a dynamic and interdependent system.

The literature on family sociology and family therapy emphasizes the importance and influence of each member of a system on other members and on the whole system. The 'health' of the family can be evaluated by examining the degree of flexibility, communication, mutuality of responsibility and sharing among family members, and therefore the health or illness of one member affects and is affected by the system as a whole (Nichols, 1984; Walsh, 1982).

Having focused on the most basic subunit of the family—the marital dyad— our study points clearly to the very high degree of mutuality between husband and wife in terms of their psychological adjustment to breast cancer and surgery. Our findings highlight the need to refer to the marital dyad when we speak about the trajectory of illness, specifically chronic illness, that the person/unit undergoes.

Medically, we describe the patient as the person who has the illness, but psychologically it is not the individual, rather the unit, that goes through illness and lives under the constant ambiguity of a new recurrence.

How much can we separate the physiological from the psychological if we aim towards cure, survival, adjustment and better quality of life? We suggest the need to change the semantics and understanding of breast cancer from the 'mastectomy patient' to the 'mastectomy couple' in order to widen our perspective and our treatment modes.

We expect, perhaps, too much of the patient who should bear her burden with fortitude, or her partner who should support and encourage her strength and competence. We would do better, we propose, to involve the mastectomy couple together in every stage of diagnosis, treatment and rehabilitation. We propose to start talking about 'the unit', 'we'/'us', and perceiving the unit as a system of responsibility in spite of the individual differentiation of each person. If social support, fighting spirit and active coping are all variables affecting the quality of life and maybe survival, then we must start under- standing and reinforcing the interaction between husband and wife (Dero- gatis, Abeloff and Melisaratos, 1979; Levy, 1984; Pettingale *et al.*, 1985). By working with the 'we' of breast cancer, we can stress and maximize the strength of the couple as a 'unit' in their coping and adaptation to a mutual chronic crisis.

REFERENCES

Baider, L., and Kaplan De-Nour, A. (1984). Couples' reactions and adjustment to mastectomy, *Int. J. Med. Psychiat.*, **14**, 265–276.
Baider, L., Rizel, S., and Kaplan De-Nour, A. (1986). Comparison of couples' adjustment to lumpectomy and mastectomy, *Gen. Hosp. Psych.*, **8**, 251–257.
Bard, M. (1952). The sequence of emotional reactions in radical mastectomy patients, *Publ. Health Rep.*, **67**, 1144–1148.
Bard, M., and Sutherland, A. M. (1977). Adaptation to radical mastectomy: The psychological impact of cancer, *Prof. Educat. Publ. Am. Canc. Soc.*, New York.
Beck, A. T., and Beamesderfer, A. (1974). Assessment of depression: The depression inventory, in *Psychological Measurement in Psychopharmacology. Modern Prob- lems in Pharmacopsychiatry* (Ed. P. Pichot), Karger, Basle.
Bloom, J. R. (1982a). Social support, accommodation to stress and adjustment to breast cancer, *Soc. Sci. Med.*, **16**, 1329–1338.

Bloom, J. R. (1982b). Social support systems and cancer: a conceptual view, in *Psychosocial Aspects of Cancer* (Eds J. Cohen, J. Cullen and R. Martin), Raven Press, New York, Chapter 14.

Chekryn, J. (1984). Cancer recurrence: personal meaning, communication and marital adjustment, *Cancer Nursing*, **7**, 491–498.

Corbin, J. M., and Strauss, A. L. (1984). Collaboration: couples working together to manage chronic illness, *Image: J. Nursing Scholarship*, **16**, 109–115.

Derogatis, L. R., Abeloff, M. D., and Melisaratos, N. (1979). Psychological coping mechanisms and survival in metastatic breast cancer, *JAMA*, **242**, 1504–1508.

Derogatis, L. R., and Lopez, M. C. (1983). PAIS and PAIS-SR—Administration scoring and procedures manual, *Clin. Psychomet. Res.*

Funch, D. P., and Mettlin, C. (1982). The role of support in the relation to recovery from breast surgery, *Soc. Sci. Med.*, **16**, 91–98.

Goldberg, R. J., and Wool, M. S. (1985). Psychotherapy for the spouses of lung cancer patients: assessment of an intervention, *Psychother. Psychos.*, **43**, 141–150.

Goldberg, R. J., Wool, M., Tull, R., *et al.* (1984). Teaching brief psychotherapy for spouses of cancer patients: use of a codable supervision format, *Psychother. Psychos.*, **41**, 12–19.

Gotay, C. C. (1984). The experience of cancer during early and advanced stages: the view of patients and their mates, *Soc. Sci. Med.*, **18**, 605–613.

Gottschalk, L. A., and Hoigard-Martin, J. (1986). The emotional impact of mastectomy, *Psych. Res.*, **17**, 153–167.

Grandstaff, N. W. (1976). The impact of breast cancer on the family, *Front. Radiat. Ther. Oncol.*, **11**, 146.

Holland, J. (1976). The clinical course of breast cancer: a psychological perspective, *Front. Radiat. Ther. Oncol.*, **11**, 133–145.

Holland, J., and Jacobs, E. (1986). Psychiatric sequelae following surgical treatment of breast cancer, *Adv. Psych. Med.*, **15**, 109–123.

Holland, J., and Mastrovito, R. (1980). Psychologic adaptation to breast cancer, *Cancer*, **46**, 1045–1052.

Hughes, J. (1982). Emotional reactions to the diagnosis and treatment of early breast cancer, *J. Psych. Res.*, **26**, 277–283.

Jamison, K. R., Wellisch, D. K., and Pasnau, R. O. (1978). Psychosocial aspects of mastectomy: the woman's perspective, *Am. J. Psych.*, **135**, 432–436.

Johnstone-Wyatt, B. G. (1981). A sexual and rehabilitative needs assessment of mastectomy couples, Doctoral dissertation, University of Pennsylvania, 1981.

Joiner, J. G., and Fisher, J. Z. (1981). Postmastectomy counseling, in *Women and Mental Health* (Eds E. Howel and M. Hayes), Basic Books, New York, pp. 411–418.

Knobf, T. M. (1986). Physical and psychologic distress associated with adjuvant chemotherapy in women with breast cancer, *J. Clin. Oncol.*, **4**, 678–684.

Levy, S. (1984). Emotions and the progression of cancer: a review, *Advances*, **1**, 10–15.

Lichtman, R. R., Wood, J. V., and Taylor, S. E. (1982). Close relationships after breast cancer, Paper presented at Am. Psych. Assoc., August 1982, Washington DC.

Lindsey, A. M., Norbeck, J. S., Carrieri, V. L., *et al.* (1981). Social support and health outcomes in postmastectomy women: a review, *Cancer Nursing*, **4**, 377–384.

Maguire, P. (1975). The psychological and social consequences of breast cancer, *Nurs. Mirror*, **140**, 540–547.

Mechanic, D. (1974). Social structure and personal adaptation: some neglected dimensions, in *Coping and Adaptation* (Eds G. V. Coelho *et al.*), Basic Books, New York, pp. 32–44.

Metzger, L. F., Rogers, T. F., and Bauman, L. J. (1983). Effects of age and marital status on emotional distress after mastectomy, *J. Psychosoc. Oncol.*, **1**, 17–33.

Meyerowitz, B. E. (1980). Psychosocial correlates of breast cancer and its treatments, *Psych. Bull.*, **87**, 108–131.

Miller, J. F. (Ed.) (1983). *Coping with Chronic Illness: Overcoming Powerlessness*, Davis, Philadelphia.

Moos, R. H., and Moos, B. S. (1981). *Family Environment Scale*, Consulting Psychologists Press, Palo Alto.

Nichols, M. (Ed.) (1984). *Family Therapy. Concepts and Methods*, Gardner Press, New York.

Pettingale, W. K., Morris, T., Greer, S., *et al.* (1985). Mental attitudes to cancer: an additional prognostic factor, *Lancet*, **1**, 750.

Plummer, E. H. (1985). Factors affecting partners' intimate reactions to mastectomy, Doctoral dissertation, California School of Psychology, Los Angeles.

Revenson, T. A., Wollman, C. A., and Felton, B. J. (1983). Social supports as stress buffers for adult cancer patients, *Psych. Med.*, **45**, 321–331.

Sabo, D., Brown, J., and Smith, C. (1986). The male role and mastectomy: support groups and men's adjustment, *J. Psychosoc. Oncol.*, **4**, 19–31.

Shanan, J. (1973). Coping behavior in the assessment of complex tasks, *Proc. 17th Int. Cong. Appl. Psych. (Liege)*, **19**, 313–321.

Shanan, J., Kaplan De-Nour, A., and Garty, I. (1976). Effects of prolonged stress on coping style in terminal renal failure patients, *J. Hum. Stress*, **2**, 19–27.

Silberfarb, P. M., Maurer, L. H., and Crouthamel, C. S. (1980). Psychosocial aspects of neoplastic disease: functional status of breast cancer patients during different treatment regimens, *Am. J. Psychiat.*, **137**, 450–455.

Spielberger, C. D., Gorsuch, R. L., and Lushen, R. E. (1970). *Manual for State Trait Anxiety Inventory*. Consulting Psychologists Press, Palo Alto.

Steinglass, P., Kaplan De-Nour, A., and Shye, S. (1985). Factors influencing psychosocial adjustment to forced geographical relocation: the Israeli withdrawal from Sinai, *Am. J. Psychiat.*, **55**, 513–529.

Taylor, S. E., Lichtman, R. R., and Wood, J. V. (1984). Attributions, beliefs about control and adjustment to breast cancer, *J. Person. Soc. Psych.*, **46**, 489–502.

Wabrek, A. J., and Wabrek, C. J. (1976). Mastectomy: sexual implications, *Primary Care*, **3**, 803.

Walsh, F. (Ed.) (1982). *Normal Family Processes*, The Guilford Press, New York.

Weisman, A., and Worden, W. J. (1977). The fallacy in postmastectomy depression, *Am. J. Med. Sci.*, **273**, 169–175.

Wellish, D. K., Jamison, K. R., and Pasnau, R. O. (1978). Psychosocial aspects of mastectomy: II. The man's perspective, *Am. J. Psychiat.*, **135**, 543–546.

Stress and Breast Cancer
Edited by C. L. Cooper
© 1988 John Wiley & Sons Ltd

Chapter 9
The Psycho-Oncologist in a Multidisciplinary Breast Treatment Center

Robert S. Hoffman
The Breast Center, Van Nuys, California, USA and Department of Psychiatry, UCLA Center for the Health Sciences, Los Angeles, USA

INTRODUCTION

The diagnosis of breast cancer confronts women and their significant others with an all too common and almost uniformly dreadful experience. Standard diagnostic and therapeutic procedures involve a series of multiple steps and a variety of physicians. Often there are numerous referrals, from the primary care provider (family practitioner, gynecologist, internist) to mammographer, back to the initial examiner, then to at least one surgeon and, more and more frequently, to a medical oncologist, radiation therapist and/or reconstructive surgeon. Second and third opinions are commonplace. These referrals, with their attendant procedures, are usually fraught with anxiety for the patient and her family. Routine operational delays prolong the agony, frequently for weeks, before a definitive diagnosis of cancer is established, which then dramatically intensifies the emotional distress. This stress is compounded by the necessity for definitive surgery (lumpectomy, axillary node dissection, or most traumatic, mastectomy) and/or radiation therapy and/or chemotherapy. Unless the patient requests psychological assistance (an uncommon occurrence) or decompensates into frank crisis, precipitating referral for psychiatric or psychological consultation (an even less common phenomenon), there is rarely any professional psychotherapeutic intervention, despite frequent manifestations of overt symptomatology. This sad state of affairs continues through the trauma of chemotherapy, the seemingly endless time of uncertainty that follows definitive treatment, the anguish of recurrence(s), and even the emotional torment that often characterizes dying from metastatic cancer.

Although initial studies failed to demonstrate a relationship between stress and breast cancer (Greer and Morris, 1975; Muslin, Gyarfas and Pieper, 1966; Schoenfeld, 1975; Snell and Graham, 1971), psychological theories about the contribution of body-image conflicts to breast cancer are controversial (Boyd, 1984), and some studies contradict the notion of significant emotional distress in breast cancer patients (Lanskey *et al.*, 1985), at least until diagnosis is known (Romsaas *et al.*, 1986), there is abundant clinical, anecdotal, empirical and academic evidence regarding the multifaceted relationship between psychological factors and treatment at all stages of breast cancer (Margolis, 1986; Watson *et al.*, 1984; Schain *et al.*, 1983, 1985; Wellisch, Silverstein and Hoffman, 1987; Sanger and Reznikoff, 1981; Steinberg, Juliano and Wise, 1985; Ashcroft, Leinster and Slade, 1985; Bartelink, Van Dam and Van Dongen, 1985; Taylor, Lichtman and Wood, 1985; Wellisch *et al.*, 1985, 1987). Multiple authors have suggested the importance of psychological factors to quality of life as well as survival for breast cancer patients and their families (Lichtman *et al.*, 1984; Vachon, Freeman and Lancee, 1985; Casolith *et al.*, 1985; Davis, 1985; Temoshok, 1986). Specific programs to implement psychosocial services for these patients have been described (Wellisch, 1984; Schover, 1986) and the beneficial uses of psychological techniques to augment medical approaches have been documented (Morrow and Morrell, 1982; Schillo-Coady, Hoffman and Silverstein, 1987). This wealth of evidence strongly suggests the potential benefit of a psycho-oncologist to a multidisciplinary team approach to the diagnosis and treatment of breast cancer.

THE BREAST CENTER

The first Breast Center opened in 1979 as part of a private medical center (Silverstein *et al.*, 1986). It was designed and decorated to provide a feeling of warmth and comfort, and staffed by a master's level oncology nurse and a master's level psychiatric nurse to assist a surgical oncologist. The center initiated a weekly academic breast cancer tumor board to which physicians, nurses and allied health professionals interested in breast cancer were invited. The original intention was to create a panel of various specialists, including cancer surgeons, reconstructive surgeons, medical oncologists, radiation therapists and psychiatrists, who would rotate coverage for new breast cancer patients and provide comprehensive care. However, this concept did not really facilitate coordinated, convenient, centralized and compassionate care.

Instead, the surgical oncologist began to refer patients to selected physicians, whose participation in, and contribution to, the Tumor Board impressed him. In addition, he arranged for a private psychiatrist from the Tumor Board group to provide supervision to the psychiatric nurse, who rendered direct supportive care to most Breast Center patients except those specifically requiring psychiatric intervention for psychopathologic decompensation.

From this consultative model, a team of private, academically oriented practitioners evolved, providing the core for a freestanding Breast Center that could actually provide comprehensive diagnosis and management of breast disease.

An entire floor of a new professional medical building adjacent to the hospital was constructed to provide a unique hospitable environment very different from traditional medical offices. The 10 000 square foot complex was designed with the latest technology and equipment available, and includes an operating suite, a psychiatric suite and an education center in addition to the usual physicians' offices, examining and consultation rooms. In contrast to the formal, often benevolently autocratic style of standard surgical practice, the center developed an informal consultative, educational and supportive approach. Patients are made to feel that they are part of an extended family. Special attention is given to speedy, efficient evaluation; entire work-ups are provided from initial examinations through thermography, ultrasonography, diaphanoscopy, mammography, needle aspiration biopsy and even definitive diagnostic biopsy (using the latest techniques including hooked wire guided biopsy) within a few days.

Once diagnosis is established, a health educator, also serving as patient advocate, guides the patient and her family through treatment, arranging and coordinating appointments for consultations with the various specialists. Patients are thoroughly informed and assisted in participating in the choice of a course of treatment most suitable to their particular biopsychosocial situations. As a result, many patients who come for second or third opinions elect to remain for treatment at the Breast Center.

THE ROLE OF THE PSYCHO-ONCOLOGIST

(a) Historical Perspective

The original physicians attending the Tumor Board included a psychiatrist with training in internal medicine and experience in family practice and emergency medicine. He was selected to supervise the first Breast Center's psychiatric nurse and provide psychiatric consultation to selected patients referred by the surgical oncologist (the first physician to work with the surgical oncologist regularly).

LR, a 44-year-old married housewife and partner in her husband's business, initially presented with a benign lump in her breast in 1979. She returned in 1981 with another lump requiring biopsy and manifested evidence of a hospital phobia. Referred for psychiatric consultation, she was able to utilize supportive intervention and undergo both biopsy and subsequent mastectomy. Later, she developed severe psychological symptoms when confronted with adjuvant chemotherapy, which she aborted after several cycles. When she developed recurrence and subsequently metastatic disease, she required further crisis psychotherapeutic intervention to overcome her reluctance to chemotherapy and was able to tolerate extensive chemotherapy with psychological support. She eventually returned home and resumed bowling and leading an active life.

The psychiatrist proved sufficiently valuable to be chosen as an integral part of the multidisciplinary Breast Center team.

As part of his developing expertise in breast cancer, the psycho-oncologist has attended breast cancer and psycho-oncology conferences, nationally and internationally, and weekly Breast Center Tumor Boards for six years, where all aspects of breast cancer, including diagnostic imaging and histopathology, are routinely presented, along with surgical, medical and radiotherapeutic issues in an educational format. He has also remained in touch with the relevant breast cancer medical literature.

At first, diagnosed breast cancer patients were offered psychiatric consultation, but almost universally declined politely while extolling the theoretical virtues of that kind of intervention for archetypal other patients who 'undoubtedly needed it', unlike themselves. However, emotional turmoil was often evident, occasionally necessitating crisis intervention and precipitating physician referral for psychiatric consultation. This prompted the routinization of automatic preoperative psychiatric consultation, initially at the time of admission to the hospital. However, the high incidence of psychologic distress during the interval between diagnosis and initiation of definitive treatment prompted provision of automatic psychiatric consultation as soon as possible after diagnosis and prior to admission. Follow-up was later provided by the psycho-oncologist to patients and family as indicated or requested between initial visit and initiation of surgical and/or medical treatment, then automatically on admission preoperatively, and postoperatively on an as-needed basis. Subsequently, routine postoperative psychological follow-up was provided by one of the teams' female psychologists. This affords the patients the opportunity to consult with a female professional and develop a broader support system. After discharge, patients may currently elect individual, marital, family or group therapy, crisis, brief or open-ended treatment, ranging from supportive and insight-oriented dynamic psychotherapy to psychopharmacotherapy to behavior modification, hypnosis, relaxation training and guided imagery. Treatment is arranged with the most appropriate member of the psychosocial support team. That team now includes two female doctors of psychology, one with extensive experience with breast cancer patients at UCLA, whose doctoral thesis involved breast cancer patients and who has published in the field (Cohen, Giuliano and Wellisch, 1984; Wellisch and Cohen, 1985), the other an ex-lumpectomy and radiation therapy patient herself (Greenberg, 1988); a female oncology nurse with a master's degree in psychiatric nursing whose master's thesis concerned the use of guided imagery with breast cancer patients (Schillo-Coady, Hoffman and Silverstein, 1987); and a female marriage and family therapist who has been counseling Breast Center patients and their families under the supervision of the psycho-oncologist for six years.

(b) Current function of the psycho-oncologist

The psycho-oncologist is director of psychosocial services, developing, providing and coordinating psychiatric treatment, education and research, as well as liaison to the Breast Center physicians, Breast Center nursing and paramedical staff, hospital nursing staff, and physicians and nurses in the community. He supervises treatment rendered by the rest of the psychiatric staff and makes final treatment decisions. It is his responsibility to provide initial consultations to both the patient and the multidisciplinary team and to inform the Tumor Board of relevant psychosocial factors pertinent to both individual cases and to general discussions of diverse aspects of breast cancer diagnosis and treatment (see Figure 1).

1. The initial consultation

If there is one crucial function central to the psycho-oncologist's role, it is the initial consultation. That is arranged to take place as soon as possible after diagnosis is established. It often involves both the patient and one or more significant other(s), like the husband, boyfriend, parent(s) (most often the mother) or sibling(s) (invariably a sister). The consultation usually lasts between one and two hours, depending on the needs and accessibility of the patient. While a range of topics are generally included, there is no rigid standard format, and the focus varies according to the most pressing issues presented. Every initial consultation includes an evaluation of the patient, including history of the patient's experience of her breast cancer, past psycho-social history (however brief), an assessment of her support system and current social milieu and a mental status examination. The small percentage of patients in crisis receive crisis intervention as rapidly as possible, often on the day of diagnosis, with supportive psychotherapy and pharmacotherapy when indicated. Anxiolytic (e.g. alprazolam) and hypnotic (e.g. triazolam) medications are the most commonly prescribed during the initial week(s) prior to admission, although the use of medication is relatively rare. Follow-up patients may be scheduled for crisis treatment but most can be managed with very brief intervention.

The overwhelming majority of patients report brief episodes (from several hours to a couple of days) of acute emotional reaction and some catharsis, followed by a period of relative calm and an emphasis on coping. They may express surprise at how 'well' they are handling their diagnosis,

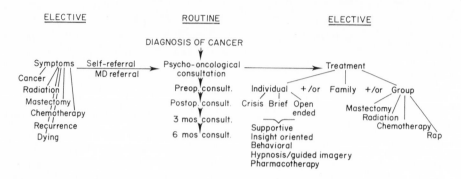

Figure 1: Psycho-oncology consultation.

frequently commenting that friends and relatives note their equanimity in the fact of adversity. The majority of patients focus on factual information and many, even though they are educated at each step of their course through diagnosis and treatment planning, pursue a better understanding by reading.

However, most do not have a clear grasp of the nature of their illness, the real meaning of statistical prognosis, or the rationale for the various treatment approaches. Therefore, the initial psycho-oncologic intervention often emphasizes education about the biology of breast cancer and its treatment. Those patients confronted with choosing between mastectomy and breast conservation are assisted by elucidation of the issues involved. Preeminent among those considerations are the distinction between systemic and local disease and the factors involved in achieving local control and reducing local recurrence rates. A discussion of statistics in general, and the statistics of breast cancer in particular, including prognostic considerations, is included. Some patients reverse their decisions, usually those having been based on misconception or incomplete understanding, even up to the last night before surgery, occasionally necessitating alterations in the surgery schedule for the next morning.

Other patients are helped to resolve conflicts about immediate versus delayed reconstruction and/or about alternative reconstructive procedures. The concept of adjuvant chemotherapy is routinely introduced and explained to disabuse patients of common predjudices and prepare them for the potential recommendation that chemotherapy be added to surgery and/or radiotherapy in order to enhance disease-free survival.

In addition to the biology of breast cancer, the psychology of breast cancer is discussed at length. A modern disease model, integrating psyche and soma, is presented including etiologic and therapeutic considerations. Patients and those close to them are given an idea of the wide range of emotional reactions they may experience themselves and may observe characterizing each other at various stages in their emotional adjustment. Psychological sequelae to breast cancer as a potentially life-threatening illness, to concerns about death and dying, to mastectomy, radiotherapy, chemotherapy and reconstructive surgery, are described, on the basis of anecdotal and empirical observations (clinical experience) and psychiatric research. Notions about the relationship between depression and the development of cancer and positive attitude and the cure of cancer are addressed. Patients are disabused of guilt feelings about causing their illnesses. An attempt is made to free them from the lonely isolation of secret 'negative thoughts and feelings' which they are afraid to acknowledge or express lest they cause recurrence or offend and provoke criticism from well-meaning but ill-informed well-wishers for whom an emphasis on positive attitude is more convenient, more hopeful and less threatening.

Both patients and their significant others are helped to distinguish between superficial reassurance and genuine support, and between coping ('I'm doing well . . . I don't cry at all') and healing. Permission and encouragement are offered to facilitate the struggle for eventual integration of the traumatic experience of breast cancer into a life of continuing emotional growth. Patients are intellectually prepared for a struggle which may well involve confrontation of denial about mortality, catharsis including profound grief and mourning, and periods of regression during which coping is at least temporarily sacrificed. (Of course those patients for whom emotional confrontation or even educational intellectualization is too threatening are not confronted with this kind of information, but are given support for their defences, especially if they are relatively primitive defenses, like blind religious faith.) Couples are introduced to the kinds of stress that relationships might encounter and approaches that might prove useful to them.

In many cases, the initial interview provides an opportunity for patients to become better informed participants in their own treatment. It also establishes an initial relationship with a member of the mental health team, who describes the many available psychosocial support services, facilitating future contact for people who might otherwise do the best they can on their own. The vast majority of patients, however skeptical they may have been about the necessity for psychiatric consultation, express gratitude for the intervention. They feel genuinely cared for and attended to, and they experience dramatic diminution in anxiety. Moreover, an initial consultation report is dictated and made available to the multidisciplinary team, which can then tailor its interactions to the emotional needs and capacities of each individual patient. Some patients are approached gingerly, out of respect for identified areas of fragility. Procedures may be modified (i.e. biopsy with local vs general anesthesia), or withheld (e.g. chemotherapy or reconstruction) when patients are unable to tolerate them emotionally.

2. Preoperative consultation

After the initial consultation, the psycho-oncologist routinely contacts those patients who are admitted (the majority) the night before surgery, except for those admitted directly to surgery in the morning (usually because their insurance company refuses to authorize preadmission). A small minority of patients present with large tumors and apparently advanced disease and are not admitted until several months of chemotherapy have been administered prior to mastectomy or iridium implantation. A very few are never admitted, having outpatient mastectomy or receiving only external beam radiation, after initial chemotherapy, without axillary node dissection. Although most patients are recompensated by the time of admission, having recovered from any transient emotional catharsis, some manifest significant anxiety, remain ambivalent about their treatment decisions or experience difficulty sleeping. The psycho-oncologist provides support and prescribes anxiolytic and/or hypnotic medication.

3. Postoperative consultation

Although patients are not seen the day of surgery because they usually manifest waxing and waning levels of consciousness, and often cannot remember events of that day, they are routinely seen the day after surgery and the day they receive the results of their axillary node dissection if those results are positive. These visits include assessment of postoperative pain, anxiety and depression. They offer the opportunity for emotional support and further education when appropriate regarding chemotherapy and/or reconstructive surgery. While postoperative consultations were originally provided by the psycho-oncologist on an as-needed basis, they are now accomplished by one of the psychologists, who alternate coverage but then follow the patients they have contacted to provide continuity of care. The psycho-oncologist is called in to assess the need for pharmacotherapy and render it when indicated, to treat pain, anxiety, depression and/or sleep disorders. Patients whose nodes are found to be positive are given special attention and followed more carefully.

When possible, spouses and children are seen for counseling while the patient is in the hospital, to educate and support them, setting the stage for ongoing involvement in the patient's life. Patients and their families are made aware of the various support services available after discharge and encouraged to participate as little or as much as is comfortable for them.

4. Post discharge

At present, participation in psychosocial support activities after discharge from the initial hospitalization is usually elective. A small percentage of patients opt for continuing individual, couple, family or group therapy. Another small group are referred for psychiatric evaluation and treatment. However, routine follow-up consultation for all patients at three and nine months is in the process of implementation. This will permit reevaluation at crucial junctures in the initial treatment or recovery phase. Those with subclinical symptoms of psychological disturbance and those whose symptoms are not apparent to other physicians providing follow-up (e.g. medical oncologist, radiation oncologist, surgical oncologist) may be captured for beneficial psychotherapeutic intervention. In addition to routine follow-up examinations, patients will be given a specially developed psychiatric questionnaire, matched with a questionnaire which will also be completed by the medical oncologist, at 6, 12, 24, 36, 48 and 60 months. These will help identify patients at high risk for emotional disturbance, who will then be scheduled for a further psychiatric evaluation.

5. Psychosocial services

Few patients elect to participate in ongoing psychosocial support. Of those who do, the majority utilize services of the Breast Center, even traveling great distances. Some already have their own therapist, others go to therapists nearer to their home if they live far from the Breast Center or to specialized cancer support centers, like the Wellness Community in Santa Monica. Occasionally, patients and their families utilize both community services and those offered by the Breast Center.

At the Breast Center, a considerable number of patients attend free, monthly, educational meetings, some regularly. The meetings begin with an hour's educational presentation by a specialist on some aspect of breast cancer. Then various oncologists, therapists and invited speakers rotate each month and address specific topics of interest, ranging from theoretical discussions about the etiology of breast cancer to demonstrations about reconstructive surgery. The more formal presentation is followed by an informal 'rap' group, led by the presenter. Special meetings are designed for husbands, couples, mothers and daughters, and other specific target populations. In addition, ongoing weekly support groups are being offered. A ten-week group guided imagery program involving anatomic and physiologic education and specific visualization has provided anxiolysis (Schillo-Coady, Hoffman and Silverstein, 1987).

An open-ended drop-in mastectomy group and a lumpectomy radiation group which patients enter at the beginning of their outpatient radiation treatment and leave after eight weeks, two weeks after radiation treatment ends, have been initiated. Chemotherapy patients are offered a ten-week long weekly 'survival style' course, offered quarterly by the young model actress who went through chemotherapy at the Breast Center and developed resources for wigs, scarves and beauty supplies and developed techniques for dressing and make-up that permitted her to work without disclosing that she was receiving an Adriamycin-containing chemotherapy regimen, even though she lost all her hair. Chemotherapy patients may also elect hypnotherapy and guided imagery, offered on an individual basis (by the psychologist with years of experience at the UCLA oncology service and in private practice), to help them manage side effects, especially anticipatory nausea and vomiting (Morrow and Morrell, 1982; Schillo-Coady, Hoffman and Silverstein, 1987). A significant number also see the psycho-oncologist for pharmacotherapeutic management of side effects and for supportive psychotherapy. The psycho-oncologist also presents intensive experiential one- and two-day long holo-tropic therapy workshops utilizing a technique developed by Stanislav Grof, MD, involving a group of about 15–25 participants, combining hyperventil-ation, evocative music and focused body work. Profound and lasting experi-ences of psychological healing have been commonly reported from these experiential group sessions.

In addition to these more specialized approaches, the Center mental health staff provides individual, marital and family therapy, supervised and coordi-nated by the psycho-oncologist.

6. Ancillary services

In addition to rendering direct treatment and supervising the treatment deliv-ered by the other team mental health professionals, the psycho-oncologist provides ongoing consultation to both team and outside physicians, formally through written report and informally by verbal contact. Currently, psycho-logical education is offered at weekly Tumor Board conferences which have contributed dramatically to raising the consciousness of those who attend regularly, including most Breast Center staff and a considerable number of health professionals from the community. A weekly conference of the medical oncologist and the mental health team has provided the opportunity for exchange of information and coordination of treatment for all patients undergoing chemotherapy at the Center. Regular psychosocial rounds with the entire staff have been difficult to sustain operationally. Liason with team paramedical staff, including nurses, and with hospital nursing staff will be continuous. A mental health professional has met weekly with the hospital nursing staff from the floor to which the Breast Center patients are admitted. Plans include weekly meetings with hospital staff most involved in the care of Breast Center patients. Liaison activities will increase when the hospital completes an inpatient unit being designed specifically for Breast Center patients who require hospitalization. That unit will be staffed by selected nurses who will provide continuity of care. Similar routine liaison conferences are being considered for Breast Center nursing staff to bring about improvement in the care of outpatients at the Center itself. The psycho-oncologist also teaches with other members of the medical staff at formal Breast Center symposia and independently when invited (Hoffman, 1987a, b; Hoffman and Schillo-Coady, 1987). Besides teaching, the psycho-oncologist develops and participates in research projects, independently and with other members of the center medical team (Silverstein *et al.*, 1986, 1987a, b; Rosser *et al.*, 1986) and with outside academicians (Eldar and Hoffman, 1987; Wellisch, Silverstein and Hoffman, 1987).

FINDINGS

Over time, close to 1000 breast cancer patients have been evaluated and treated by the psycho-oncologist, a growing fraction of these also by other members of the expanding psychosocial support team.

About fifteen to twenty breast cancer patients at various stages of the disease are in ongoing treatment with the psyco-oncologist at any one time, and he performs an average of two to three consultations per week on newly diagnosed patients.

Besides patients who seek psychological assistance, others are referred for counseling, support or treatment with psychotropic medication, most often by the medical oncologist but also by the team's surgical and radiation oncologists, the reconstructive surgeon and outside physicians. Patients have traveled from San Diego, Newport Beach, Apple Valley, Santa Barbara, Bakersfield and Santa Maria, California as well as from Scottsdale, Arizona for ongoing psychiatric treatment on an occasional to regular weekly basis. Those who come from the greatest distances usually coordinate their visits with appointments to see other Breast Center physicians. Some patients come for one visit, others up to several times per week for years. Most patients have required minimal, mostly prophylactic care. Some have required crisis intervention.

CM, a 39-year-old married professional, was seen in crisis intervention on the day she received her diagnosis, in a state of near hysteria. She initially fled the psycho-oncologist's waiting room on the pretext that she had been mistreated by the secretary. Coaxed back for an initial interview, she was able to utilize the opportunity for catharsis and support, and calmed down considerably. She returned for several sessions prior to medical treatment, and was initially prescribed anxiolytic medication (Xanax and alprazolam) before her admission for axillary node dissection and iridium implantation. After a temporary hiatus, she returned for counseling without medication on an ongoing outpatient basis to deal with exacerbation of preexisting marital problems, among other issues.

One decompensated sufficiently to prompt relatively brief psychiatric hospitalization.

RC, a 33-year-old insurance saleswoman and mother of a three-year-old daughter, married to a psychologist, with a history of one recent prior psychiatric hospitalization for suicidal depression, suffered a florid psychotic decompensation during her admission for mastectomy. She was psychiatrically hospitalized for several weeks and treated with neuroleptic medication (thiothixene). Recompensation was rapid. Although her ERA and PRA were negative and she would otherwise have been encouraged to undergo chemotherapy, despite negative axillary lymph nodes, chemotherapy was withheld in light of her fragile mental status. The patient then returned for individual therapy biweekly augmented by weekly conjoint therapy with her husband. Psychotropic medication was rapidly tapered. Her progress was dramatic. She subsequently endured chemotherapy for an inflammatory carcinoma in the contralateral breast without any evidence of psychological decompensation. After a period of disease-free survival, during which she experienced significant personal growth and reported improved quality of life, she developed brain metastases and underwent radiotherapy. She did not evidence any major emotional symptomatology through her terminal period. On the contrary, her emotional strength surprised and impressed the entire staff, who had come to know her well and to have great affection for her.

Occasionally, patients who initially appear psychologically healthy subsequently decompensate, disclosing prior history of major psychological disturbance.

JH presented as a 46-year-old divorced unemployed ex-legal secretary at the time of her axillary node dissection prior to radiation therapy. She appeared to be dealing with her situation in an emotionally appropriate, resourceful way. However, she was later referred for psychotherapy after her radiation treatment because she was decompensating. She revealed problems with her aged, ailing mother, with an alcoholic boyfriend, and a history of her own long-standing alcoholism. She was detoxified with chlorazepate as an outpatient but failed to appear for follow-up appointments until she reappeared at the Breast Center with a contralateral primary breast cancer. She returned inebriated and required detoxification and support to undergo a second course of cancer treatment. She was seen in psychotherapy for a period of time, but two years later required admission to the medical center on a 72-hour hold for suicidal depression after an overdose with her mother's sleeping pills. She reported having been drinking heavily for two months after 18 months of sobriety, and having been in jail for repeatedly driving under the influence of alcohol. She was again detoxified with chlorazepate and followed in outpatient therapy by the counselor with medical supervision from the psycho-oncologist.

Patients seek treatment at various times during their course for a multiplicity of reasons.

LF, a 44-year-old divorced administrator, referred herself for psychotherapy eight years after her mastectomy when she became convinced that recurrent symptoms in the area of her reconstruction were somatizations of unresolved emotional conflicts regarding her mastectomy.

JK, a 49-year-old recently remarried woman at the time she came for consultation, requested assistance in making a decision regarding reconstruction, which she wanted but her new husband opposed. She disclosed that her first husband, to whom she had been very unhappily married for many years (during which she was continually ill with migraine headaches and pancreatitis, finally necessitating a subtotal gastrectomy), had left her soon after her mastectomy. She went through a year of chemotherapy alone, then reentered the social world with one breast and, to her amazement, found a man who genuinely loved her and treated her kindly, in stark contrast to her first husband's self-involved, cold indifference. While struggling in brief therapy with her decision to proceed with reconstruction, the patient was confronted with her 52-year-old second husband's sudden death, almost before her eyes, of a heart attack. This precipitated crisis psychotherapeutic intervention, during which the patient revealed chronic dependence on multiple narcotic analgesics, major and minor tranquilizers, hypnotics, and antidepressants all for headaches. She then entered long-term treatment, combining dynamic and supportive insight therapy with pharmacotherapy. Although she was convinced that she was condemned to spend the rest of her life single, she did undergo reconstructive surgery. Not long after, she met a man with whom she fell in love. Therapy helped her transition from dating to marriage, and to work through many difficult marital conflicts that threatened to destroy the most fulfilling relationship of her life. In addition, after unsuccessful trials of chiropractic, acupuncture, temporal–mandibular joint treatment and biofeedback, as well as virtually every medication used to treat migraine headaches, alone and in combination, her headaches were finally controlled by a monoamine oxidase inhibitor (phenelzine), dramatically changing her experience of her daily life.

Often couples come for treatment, sometimes families, occasionally spouses by themselves, and least often, children alone.

BK, a 33-year-old married bookkeeper and mother of a two-year-old son initially presented after mastectomy and during adjuvant chemotherapy with an Adriamycin-containing regimen. Having developed her first lump when pregnant, the patient had been told that there was no problem in her breast by her obstetrician. Later, the lump enlarged and a check-up disclosed evidence of a cancer, precipitating terror in the patient, especially regarding chemotherapy. Psychiatric evaluation revealed evidence of a long-standing underlying depression, a turbulent marriage to a depressed obsessive–compulsive computer repairman (whom she met in a psychiatric hospital at age nineteen after his suicide attempt while she was being treated with 30–40 mg of trifluoperazine per day), and a history of recent increasing financial difficulty. Initial psychiatric diagnosis included an adjustment disorder with mixed emotional features, superimposed on a narcissistic personality with borderline features. Weekly conjoint therapy, alternating with individual therapy for both the patient and her husband, enabled her to tolerate debilitating chemotherapy and her husband to refrain from actively sabotaging her care. By the end of her chemotherapy, she decided to separate from her well-meaning but emotionally inadequate and insufficiently supportive husband, return to school and terminate her psychotherapy.

RF, a 35-year-old married male and father of a little girl, entered psychotherapy by himself because he wanted to save a floundering marriage seriously threatened by his inability to deal with his wife's reaction to her breast cancer. After a year of individual therapy, he was able to dedicate himself fully to strengthening his marriage.

MMcA, a 35-year-old physician's wife and mother of two, came for help to deal with her mother's breast cancer. Born when her mother was only sixteen years old, she remained unusually close to her mother even after graduation from college and marriage. The mother's cancer did not significantly emotionally traumatize the cancer patient but terrified the daughter. When the mother resumed smoking and the daughter discovered this clandestine behavior, the daughter developed overt symptomatology with anxiety, obsessive ruminations, insomnia, depressed mood and emotional lability. She presented describing herself as 'hysterical', dependent on and furious with her mother. After initial pharmacotherapy with a minor tranquilizer (alprazolam), she underwent weekly insight-oriented brief psychotherapy, lasting several months. She regained her equanimity and resolved her dependency on her mother.

Patients enter therapy to deal with cancerphobia, and chemotherapy side effects.

BG, a 41-year-old single white female professional publisher with a history of Hodgkin's disease as a teenager, entered long-term analytically oriented therapy to deal with long-standing cancerphobia which was exacerbated with a diagnosis of breast cancer to the point that she became preoccupied with death and seriously depressed.

SH, a 33-year-old married model and actress, entered treatment to help her through her Adriamycin-containing adjuvant chemotherapy regimen. Despite hair loss, she was able to work with a wig, to tolerate chemotherapy side effects, with the help of guided imagery and combinations of anti-emetic medications, and to improve a marriage threatened by the stress of her illness, with the help of marital counseling. She went on to develop a training program for chemotherapy patients to help them feel attractive through the use of wigs, scarves and make-up.

Adjuvant chemotherapy patients represent the largest contingency receiving some form of ongoing ancillary care, usually throughout the six to twelve months of their chemotherapy treatments.

EJ, a 37-year-old married school teacher and dancer who underwent lumpectomy and X-ray treatment for a small carcinoma, returned five years later with a contralateral breast cancer requiring a modified radical mastectomy followed by an Adriamycin-containing regimen of adjuvant chemotherapy, after meticulous follow-up in her geographical area failed to detect the second cancer in an early stage. She felt terribly guilty because her friends told her that she must have brought the cancer on herself. She revealed that she had been sexually molested and brutalized by alcoholic parents, and disclosed a subsequent history of polymorphous perverse sexual activity. A combination of analytically oriented psychotherapy and experiential treatment with Grof breathing produced dramatic personal growth and resolution of long-standing emotional conflicts.

Recurrence and preterminal disease commonly precipitate self-referral.

PN, a 47-year-old married housewife and mother of grown children, presented to the medical oncologist severely depressed at the time of her first recurrence. Referred for psychiatric evaluation, she was initially treated with tricyclic antidepressant medication (amitriptyline) for a major depressive disorder with suicidal ideation. She also entered weekly analytically-oriented insight psychotherapy and made a remarkably rapid recovery, not only overcoming her debilitating, vegetative depression in a matter of two months, but proceeding to significant emotional growth and alteration in a long-standing unfulfilling marriage.

Patients and their families often seek help to deal with the issues of death and dying. This is usually managed by the psycho-oncologist. Medication management for control of pain, anxiety and depression is coordinated by the medical and psycho-oncologists, both of whom make home visits, attend patients at hospices, and provide daily care to dying hospitalized patients.

ED, an intelligent educated 46-year-old married real estate entrepreneur, was initially seen at the time her breast cancer was diagnosed. She had her own therapist, a behaviorist, who had been treating her for a phobia, and she declined further support. Years later, when she was confronted with progressive metastatic disease, she requested further psychiatric consultation. At that time, she revealed that her therapist, a female clinical psychologist at a local university medical center, had strongly dissuaded her from pursuing treatment by the Breast Center psychiatrist because a psychiatrist would burden her with irrelevant analysis of her childhood and her relationship with her mother, according to the psychologist. The bahaviorist reassured the patient repeatedly over the years that she was psychologically healthy, and declined to treat her, electing instead to be her friend but gradually disappearing from her life. At the same time, the patient's husband insisted that a positive attitude would cure her, and that any 'negative' emotions, like fear, might contribute to recurrence. This belief was strongly reinforced by the patient's new support group, an analog of Jews For Jesus, to whom the patient and her husband turned for faith and healing. After church healers had repeatedly prayed for the patient and laid on hands, the patient was unable to suppress her 'negative' feelings like despair and terror, and tentatively asked the Breast Center psychiatrist for help. She then embarked on outpatient psychotherapy, augmented by family therapy. This eventuated in home hospice care with psychopharmacotherapeutic intervention to manage her pain, depression and anxiety, until she died. Both her husband and her daughter received psychological support through the entire terminal phase of her illness, and her daughter continued in crisis therapy for a brief period after her mother's death.

MJ, initially presented as a 45-year-old married, retired teacher, manager of her family's successful restaurant chain and mother of two troubled adopted children. She underwent a modified radical mastectomy and abdominal flap reconstructive surgery, which failed. Terrified, she attempted to handle her emotional distress intellectually as she had always handled emotional issues. However, she remained terrified, but, with psychotherapeutic intervention, was able to cope with severe family problems. Subsequently, she valiantly suffered through extremely painful metastatic disease including brain metastases, and severely toxic chemotherapy, which she took as much to preserve hope for herself as to treat her cancer. Finally, she came to peace with herself, was able to face death, said goodbye to her family and elected a course of analgesia that rendered her pain-free until she died. Both her husband and her children were assisted with understanding and accepting her condition as it evolved, were guided through their interactions with her, and were supported through anticipatory grief prior to her demise.

A typical recent week in the psycho-oncologist's practice included, besides three initial consultations for newly diagnosed patients (and ongoing treatment of women at all stages of breast cancer), a day in which four inpatient consultations were requested by the medical oncologist.

A preterminal woman with brain metastases requiring steroids to control cerebral edema was increasingly paranoid and tormenting her husband and children with accusations of abandonment. Although the family was very biased against psychiatry as hocus-pocus for crazy people, they were sufficiently distraught to accept any help proferred and grateful when treatment with low-dose neuroleptic medication (haloperidol) produced a dramatic reversal within 24 hours, reuniting them with the patient.

A chronically borderline patient with a history of micropsychotic paranoid episodes became floridly psychotic, precipitating urgent requests from nursing to transfer the patient to psychiatry and treat her with a major tranquilizer. However, the patient, hospitalized to manage her chronic pain syndrome, was suffering from a central anitcholinergic syndrome precipitated by a combination of drugs and promptly recompensated after her medication, including narcotic analgesics, was discontinued.

A 39-year-old divorced mother of two young children with advanced metastatic disease, manifesting waxing and waning levels of consciousness, required little personal assistance, but her children, who had no other family, needed emotional support.

A 55-year-old woman dying with cancer in her lungs benefited from some support and reassurance that she was facing reality appropriately. Her oncologist also needed reassurance that there was no covert depression requiring any more invasive psychiatric intervention.

The most common issues presented include loss of innocence and rupture of denial manifested as mourning, fear of recurrence, fear of death, alteration of body image, and loss of a sense of wholeness, especially for mastectomy patients. Other frequent problems involve chemotherapy toxicity and marital and family stress.

The most common psychopathologic diagnoses represented include adjustment disorders with depressed mood and with mixed emotional features, and dysthymic disorders. There have been several patients with major depressive disorders, several with toxic psychoses, and one with a functional psychotic decompensation requiring psychiatric hospitalization. A considerable minority require medication, most often relatively briefly for crisis levels of anxiety and transient insomnia, less often for vegetative depression, for chemotherapy side effects and for cancer-related pain.

Peaks in the incidence of psychological distress occur after diagnosis, at the conclusion of radiation treatment and chemotherapy, about six months to one year after mastectomy, at the time when recurrences are diagnosed, and at the time when patients become preterminal. The frequency and intensity of symptoms of emotional decompensation seem to be ameliorated dramatically by prophylactic and therapeutic psychosocial intervention. In addition, treatment choices have been altered (e.g. from mastectomy to conservation and *vice versa*), sometimes (literally) at the eleventh hour (the night before surgery) on the basis of psychiatric intervention.

Of course patients respond individually, usually in characterologically consistent fashion. Cultural and religious belief systems, coexisting psychological stressors, availability of a genuine support network and preexisting historical, situational and characterological factors play a role in determining psychological response and accessibility to therapeutic intervention.

As a rule, patients strive to cope, most often utilizing intellectualization, displacement, minimization and denial to avoid confrontation and expression of potentially overwhelming feelings. They consider themselves to be doing well if they don't cry or worry. Doing defenses (keeping occupied) are commonly employed. Many believe that a positive attitude will help them to heal, and that 'negative' thoughts and feelings (often those most appropriate to their psychological if not biological reality, like fear, anger and sadness) can cause cancer to recur. Therefore, they terrify themselves when they experience their true feelings and strive to suppress and control them.

This suppression of feelings is usually promoted by friends and relatives, for whom unpleasant emotional expressions are threatening and inconvenient. Feeling impotent, these well-meaning acquaintances attempt to provide support through reassurance and preach the virtues of positivity, ignoring or lecturing against the expression of negative emotions. When they do not actively avoid the patients, as friends often do, the significant others, like spouses, parents and children, usually concentrate on being helpful to the identified victims, avoiding their own feelings and the degree to which the patient's illness constitutes a serious stressor in their lives. Boyfriends may find excuses to terminate their involvement with patients—husbands rarely do, especially in strong, longstanding marriages.

Many routine findings confirm commonsense expectations. For example, mastectomy patients are more likely to experience significant emotional distress than radiation therapy patients, and chemotherapy patients are most likely to seek assistance, especially if their chemotherapy regimen includes Adriamycin or other severely toxic drugs. Mastectomy patients often complain of loss of a sense of wholeness, difficulty adapting to altered body image and problems with sexual adjustment. Sometimes patients focus on mastectomy, displacing their attention from more threatening issues of metastasis and death.

The frequency and intensity of psychological symptoms reported by mastectomy patients is dramatically curtailed by reconstructive surgery. However, complications of reconstructive surgery lead to a surprising number of emotional complaints. Radiotherapy patients are often able to avoid significant emotional distress, resurrecting denial rapidly, a defensive maneuver much more difficult for mastectomy patients even after reconstruction. Chemotherapy patients focus on day-to-day difficulties, often as if protected from recurrence during the period of the chemotherapy, then frequently become more symptomatic when the chemotherapy ends. This is much less common for those patients in psychotherapy during their chemotherapy, who are likely to celebrate the end of chemotherapy and leave their psychotherapy soon after the chemotherapy ends.

Despite the preponderance of expected reactions, some common findings are conterintuitive. For example, when couples have a history of antecedent strife, the patients are more likely to precipitate separation and divorce than the spouses. Although a few husbands have reacted to the added stress of the cancer by leaving their wives, the overwhelming majority have tried to sustain their marriages, usually recognising the previously devalued or ignored virtues of the spouse (patient) whose life is threatened, sometimes avoiding the guilt of abandoning someone in distress. Wives, on the other hand, frequently find their non-supportive or 'defective' (i.e. alcoholic, unfaithful, absent, etc.) husbands' behaviors intolerable, where they had previously rationalized or otherwise managed to suffer them. Occasionally the patients themselves consciously choose to remain in relationships they acknowledge as unsatisfactory because of their dependency needs and their insecurity about their own ability to survive alone or to improve upon their predicaments, especially if they feel that their cancer makes them undesirable. This is more often an issue with those mastectomy patients who feel mutilated.

Mastectomy patients are also likely to fear loss of their partners' sexual interest, despite verbalized reassurance from the majority of their lovers. They may believe that their husbands feel obliged to reassure them but privately find them less attractive. Interestingly, the men usually do not anticipate major sexual problems when questioned privately (although one with prior sexual problems expressed fear of impotence) and rarely experienced sexual disability. (For the most part they find a way to circumvent the absent breast.) It is the patients who, feeling unattractive, even in the face of their lovers' desire, more often experience difficulty feeling sexy enough to permit or enjoy sex until they achieve some psychological resolution.

Another paradoxical finding contradicts the general assumption that older women more often prefer mastectomy. In fact, they are as likely to want to save their breasts as younger patients, but as a group do find the mastectomy less threatening and less traumatic when it is medically advisable. However, of the small percentage of women who insist upon saving their breasts despite having been informed that mastectomy is medically indicated, an approximately equal number are elderly. The older women are more often fatalistic, the younger more often fearful of long-term effects of radiation or of psychosocial and psychosexual consequences of mastectomy. Older patients are also less likely to elect reconstructive surgery.

In contradiction to the inconclusive findings reported in the literature, the greatest majority of breast cancer patients seen at the Breast Center do share certain personality characteristics. Rarely are these classically passive, dependent or hypochondriacal women. Almost all the patients describe themselves, and are described by their relatives, as people who find it much easier to take care of other people than to allow anyone to take care of them. They tend to be more active than passive and are often competent, conscientious copers who control their feelings. They are unlikely to have integrated their dependency needs into their personalities. If anything, they overcompensate for their dependency needs, which may be prominent but masked.

Despite these generalizations, every breast cancer patient is unique when all pertinent variables are taken into account. There is no standard approach applicable to all patients. Where confrontation and catharsis may benefit some, they may precipitate decompensation in others for whom support of denial or other defenses, even primitive ones, is preferable. The highest (but not always achievable) goal of psychotherapeutic intervention is promotion of psychological healing, even more than the maintenance of coping and baseline functioning. This may involve regression in the service of the ego. Like recovery from any serious psychic injury, genuine recovery from a breast cancer experience occurs in stages, over time, leading to adaptation and, optimally, to integration of the experience, even to psychological growth. It is not uncommon for breast cancer patients eventually to express the conviction that the cancer experience prompted reprioritization of values, recognition of previously ignored but precious aspects of life, and dramatic improvement in the quality of everyday life. This process is facilitated by therapy which encourages and supports the authentic experience and expression of inconvenient and unwelcome feelings generated by the cancer, including terror, anguish, grief, even hopelessness, helplessness, and transient suicidal despair. However, many patients cannot tolerate painful, growth-promoting treatment and may achieve maintenance of function or minimize disintegration, with support for preexisting defenses and ego assets. Patients often benefit from inclusion of one or more significant others in their supportive treatment program.

FUTURE GOALS

Premier among the psycho-oncologist's priorities is improvement in routine follow-up, currently elective. This is planned through initiation of questionnaires to be self-administered and concurrently administered by the oncologist at specific intervals over a period of five years. Questionnaires will be augmented by several recommended standard follow-up psychosocial interviews in the first year.

In addition, there are plans to increase contact between staff members and to provide greater opportunity for coordination of care. Psychosocial research will be routinized with the availability of computerized data from a newly developed psychosocial database and from the questionnaires.

Areas for potential development by the psycho-oncologist that have not been addressed but remain relevant nonetheless, include formal measures to deal with staff burnout and routinization of family contact, at least initially, with spouses and children to provide baseline education and support.

CONCLUSION

A multidisciplinary academically oriented team approach to the diagnosis and treatment of breast disease has been developed and refined in the private sector over the past seven years. The team includes a psycho-oncologist with training and experience in medicine, as well as broad experience in psychiatry, including consultation–liaison psychiatry. The psycho-oncologist has pursued further training in the medical and psychiatric aspects of breast cancer by attending weekly educational tumor board meetings, national and international conferences, and by keeping abreast of the relevant literature.

During the past seven years, the role of psycho-oncologist has evolved from supervision of a psychiatric nurse and occasional elective consultation to a multiplicity of organizational, supervisorial, educational, investigative and therapeutic endeavors. The psycho-oncologist plays a crucial role, integral to the provision of humane, holistic care of breast cancer patients and their families.

REFERENCES

Ashcroft, J. J., Leinster, S. J., and Slade, P. (1985). Breast cancer: Patient choice of treatment: Preliminary communication, *J. Roy. Soc. Med.*, **78**, 43–46.

Bartelink, H., Van Dam, F., and Van Dongen, J. (1985). Psychological effects of breast conserving therapy in comparison with radical mastectomy, *Rad. Onc. Biol. Phys.*, **11**, 381–385.

Boyd, P. (1948). *The Silent Wound*, Addison Wesley, Reading, MA.

Casolith, B., Lusk, E., Strouse, T., Miller, D., Brown, L., and Cross, P. (1985). *Cancer*, **55**, 72–76.

Cohen, R. S., Giuliano, A. E., and Wellisch, D. K. (1984). Comparison of lumpectomy versus mastectomy patients: psychological, attitudinal and social impact, *Proc. Am. Soc. Clin. Oncol.*, May 1984, p. 72.

Davis, H. (1985). *Texas Med.*, **81**, 49–52.

Eldar, A., and Hoffman, R. S. (1987). Self-esteem of women after mastectomy, lumpectomy or non-breast cancer surgery, Proceedings of the International Symposium on Breast Cancer, New Delhi, January 1987.

Greenberg, M. (1988). *Invisible Scars: A Guide to the Emotional Impact of Breast Cancer.* Walker & Co.

Greer, S., and Morris, T. (1975). Psychological attributes of women who develop breast cancer: A controlled study, *J. Psychosom. Res.*, **19**, 147–53.

Hoffman, R. S. (1987a). The role of the psycho-oncologist in a multi-disciplinary breast cancer treatment center, Proceedings of the International Symposium on Breast Cancer, New Delhi, January 1987.

Hoffman, R. S. (1987b). Observations of a clinical psycho-oncologist. Proceedings of the International Symposium on Breast Cancer, New Delhi, January 1987.

Hoffman, R. S., and Schillo-Coady, L. (1987). The effect of a guided imagery program on anxiety in breast cancer patients. Proceedings of the International Symposium on Breast Cancer, New Delhi, January 1987.

Lanskey, S., List, M., Herrmann, C., Ets-Hokin, E., Das Gupta, T., Wilbanks, G., and Hendrickson, F. (1985). Absence of major depressive disorder in female cancer patients, *J. Clin. Oncol.*, **3**, No. 11.

Lichtman, R., Taylor, S., Wood, J., Bluming, A., Dosik, G., and Leibowitz, R. (1984). Relations with children after breast cancer: The mother–daughter relationship at risk, *J. Psychosoc. Oncol.*, **2** (3–4), Fall/Winter.

Margolis, G. (1986). 139th American Psychiatric Association Annual Meeting, May 1986.

Morrow, G., and Morrell, C. (1982). Behavioral treatment for the anticipatory nausea and vomiting induced by cancer chemotherapy, *New Eng. J. Med.*, December 9, **307**, 1476.

Muslin, H., Gyarfas, K., and Pieper, W. (1966). Separation experience and cancer of the breast. *Ann. NY Acad. Sci.*, **125**, 802–806.

Romsaas, E., Maleck, J., Gavenkoski, B., Trump, D., and Wolberg, W. (1986). Psychological distress among women with breast problems, *Cancer*, **57**, 890–895.

Rosser, R., Silverstein, M. J., Gamagami, P., Gearson, E., Colburn, W., Handel, N., Waisman, J., Lewinski, B., Fingerhut, A., and Hoffman, R. S. (1986). Intraductal breast carcinoma: What constitutes adequate treatment. In: *Fundamental Problems in Breast Cancer*, The Hague, Martinus Nijhoff.

Sanger, C. K., and Reznikoff, M. (1981). A comparison of the psychological effects of breast saving procedures with the modified radical mastectomy, *Cancer*, **48**, 2341–2346.

Schain, W., Edwards, B., Gorrel, C., de Moss, E., Lippman, M., Gerber, L., and Lichter, A. (1983). Psychosocial and physical outcomes of primary breast cancer therapy: Mastectomy versus excisional biopsy and irradiation, *Breast Cancer Res. Treatment*, **3**, 377–382.

Schain, W., Wellisch, D., Pasnau, R., and Landsverk, J. (1985). The sooner the better: A study of psychological factors in women undergoing immediate versus delayed breast reconstruction, *Am. J. Psychiat.*, **142**, 1.

Schover, L. (1986). Proceedings of the American Cancer Society 28th Writers' Seminar, 1986.

Schillo-Coady, L., Hoffman, R. S., and Silverstein, M. J. (1987). The effects of the visualization program on anxiety in breast cancer patients, Submitted for publication.

Schoenfeld, J. (1975). Psychological and life experience differences between Israeli women with benign and cancerous breast lesions, *J. Psychosom. Res.*, **19**, 229–234.

Silverstein, M. J., Gamagami, P., Rosser, R., Gearson, E., Colburn, W., Handel, N., Waisman, J., Lewinski, B., Fingerhut, A., and Hoffman, R. S. (1986). Finding earlier non-palpable breast cancers using hooked wire directed biopsy and a modified overpenetrated mammographic technique. In: *Fundamental Problems in Breast Cancer*, The Hague, Martinus Nijhoff.

Silverstein, M. J., Gamagami, P., Rosser, R., Gearson, E., Colburn, W., Handel, N., Waisman, J., Lewinski, B., Fingerhut, A., and Hoffman, R. S. (1987b). Hooked wire directed biopsy: 653 consecutive cases, *Cancer*, **59**, 715–722.

Silverstein, M. J., Handel, N., Hoffman, R. S., Waisman, J., Rosser, R., Gamagami, P., Gearson, E., Colburn, W., Waisman, E., Lewinski, B., and Fingerhut, A. (1986). *The Breast Center: A Multi-Disciplinary Model in Fundamental Problems in Breast Cancer*, in press.

Silverstein, M. J., Rosser, R., Gearson, E., Waisman, J., Gamagami, P., Hoffman, R. S., Fingerhut, A., Lewinski, B., Colburn, W., and Handel, N. (1987a). Axillary lymph node dissection for intraductal breast carcinoma: Is it indicated? *Cancer*, **59**, 1819–1824.

Snell, L., and Graham, S. (1971). Social trauma as related to cancer of the breast, *Brit. J. Cancer*, **25**, 721–734.

Steinberg, M., Juliano, M., and Wise, L. (1985). Psychological outcome of lumpectomy versus mastectomy in the treatment of breast cancer, *Am. J. Psychiat.*, **142**(1), 34–39.

Taylor, S. E., Lichtman, R. D., and Wodd, J. (1985). Illness related and treatment related factors and psychological adjustment to breast cancer, *Cancer*, **55**, 2506–2513.

Temoshok, L. (1986). Proceedings of the American Cancer Society 28th Writers' Seminar, 1986.

Vachon, M., Freeman, S., and Lancee, W. (1985). *Proc. Can. Psychiat. Assoc.*, **1985**.

Watson, M., Greer, S., Blake, S., and Schrapnell, K. (1984). Reaction to a diagnosis of breast cancer: Relationship between denial, delay and rates of psychological morbidity, *Cancer*, **53**, 2008–2012.

Wellisch, D. (1984). Implementation of psychosocial services in managing emotional stress, *Cancer*, **53**, 828–832.

Wellisch, D. K., and Cohen, R. S. (1985). *Psychological Aspects of Cancer in Cancer Treatment*, 2nd edn (Ed. C. M. Haskell), W. B. Saunders Co., Philadelphia.

Wellisch, D. K., Schain, W. S., Noone, B. R., and Little, J. W. (1985). Psychosocial correlates of immediate versus delayed reconstruction of the breast, *Plastic Reconstruct. Surg.*, **76** (5), 713–718.

Wellisch, D. K., Schain, W. S., Noone, B. R., and Little, J. W. (1987). The psychological contribution of nipple addition in breast reconstruction, *Plastic Reconstruct. Surg.*, in press.

Wellisch, D., Silverstein, M. J., and Hoffman, R. S. (1987). Psychosocial outcomes of breast cancer therapies: Lumpectomy versus mastectomy with and without breast reconstruction, Submitted for publication.

ROLE OF THE PSYCHO-ONCOLOGIST

I   Director of psychosocial services

   A   Supervision and coordination of mental health team activities

   B   Liaison

     1   To Breast Center staff

     2   To community physicians

   C   Program development

II Education
   A Patients
      1 Consultations
      2 'Rap' group education meetings
   B Families
   C Health professionals
      1 Tumor Board
      2 Seminars, conferences
         (a) Breast Center sponsored
         (b) Local, national, international

III Treatment
   A Psychotherapy
      1 Individual
         (a) Crisis
         (b) Brief Rx
         (c) Open-ended
            (i) supportive
            (ii) insight-oriented
            (iii) behavioral
            (iv) problem-solving
            (v) marital
            (vi) family
   B Pharmacotherapy
      1 Anxiolytic
      2 Antidepressant
      3 Hypnotic
      4 Analgesic
      5 Chemotherapy side-effects management

IV Consultation
   A Breast Center MDs
      1 Written
      2 Verbal
   B Community MDs
      1 Written
      2 Verbal

V Clinical research
   A Development
   B Conduct

Section Six
Methodological Considerations in Research

Stress and Breast Cancer
Edited by C. L. Cooper
© 1988 John Wiley & Sons Ltd

Chapter 10
Methodological Considerations in Studying the Stress–Illness Connection in Women with Breast Cancer

David F. Cella
Department of Psychology and Social Sciences, Rush Presbyterian/St Luke's Medical Center, Chicago, USA
and
Jimmie C. Holland
Memorial Sloan-Kettering Cancer Center, New York, USA

INTRODUCTION

For the past fifteen years, there has been a growing interest in the application of psychoneuroimmunology to patients with cancer. The idea that mental attitude can alter cancer risk and survival via some mediating neuroimmunological mechanism has been promoted for some time. In fact, Galen observed in the second century that breast cancer in women was associated with melancholia (Cox and MacKay, 1982; Greer and Morris, 1978). However, only within the past decade, with methodological developments in immunology, psychology and psychiatry, have there been convincing empirical data to substantiate this view (Ader, 1981; Levy, 1985). In a review article, Fox (1983) concluded that the effect of psychological factors upon cancer *incidence* is likely to be small. However, their effect upon cancer *prognosis*, or progression of existing disease, is probably stronger. After reviewing hundreds of studies, Sklar and Anisman (1981) concluded: 'although there appears to be a correlation between tumor growth and psychological factors in humans, causal relations between these variables remain to be demonstrated' (p. 374). Such demonstration can only be convincingly accomplished via prospective epidemiological studies and laboratory studies which combine psychological assessment and immunological assessment (e.g. Levy *et al.*, 1985).

If behavioral/psychological factors have a causal impact upon cancer, the impact is likely to be greatest on the *progression of slow-growing tumors*, because they are under at least partial control of endogenous hormonal or immunological factors (Levy, 1985). Such factors are known to be mediated directly and indirectly by the central nervous system (Ader, 1981). The question of whether there is a causal link between psychological factors and the immune system, mediated by endocrine or neuroendocrine alterations, is a general one in that it applies not only to cancer but to virtually all diseases. The general link between stress and immunity, at both the humoral and cell-mediated level, has been extensively studied. In a review of human studies of the relationship of psychosocial factors and the immune response, Jemmott and Locke (1984) concluded that although many studies are methodologically flawed, the bulk of the evidence confirms the view that psychosocial factors influence immunity. Again, however, they caution against the temptation to infer too much support from correlational studies which simply document an association.

Of human cancers that have been studied, breast cancer is among the sites which have received the most attention. Breast cancer is clearly a hormone-dependent malignancy which is subject to long periods of quiescence and later reemergence. Also, along with carcinoma of the lung, it is the leading cause of death due to malignancy in women. Therefore, breast cancer has commonly been identified as a good target for successful behavioral interventions to reduce risk and enhance treatment response.

Before leaping into a discussion of advances in psychoneuroimmunology and breast cancer, it is important to note that many studies have *failed* to detect an influence of psychological factors upon disease incidence and progression. These too must be reckoned with whenever one tries to determine the current state of knowledge in the area. Some studies have actually contradicted other reports that had supported an immune-modulating hypothesis. Others have simply yielded negative results. This chapter will review a selected subset of these studies, those dealing with carcinoma of the breast, in an effort to distinguish solid empirical evidence from study data that are misleading and may serve to exaggerate the extent of the stress–illness connection in breast carcinoma. The focus will be on studies of the stress–illness connection in women with breast cancer, although many of the principles could conceivably be generalized to other forms of cancer or even to the general link between stress and illness.

This chapter does not cover the hypothesized biological mechanisms associated with the link between stress and disease onset or progression: those mechanisms are discussed elsewhere in this book. Nor does this chapter emphasize the case for promoting positive attitudes in cancer patients, though indeed a case can be made: that too has been covered elsewhere in the book. The focus of this chapter is on the methodology of existing studies, with particular emphasis on limitations in design and interpretation of results. Hopefully, such a focus can lead to recommendations for future research.

Breast cancer has a tremendous impact upon a woman's psychological, social and sexual adjustment. This chapter will only address this issue from the standpoint of how these changes in adjustment might be associated with later promotion or inhibition of tumor growth. No claim is made as to which event is preexisting: distress or tumor response. There is an obvious problem of determining causality in this circular situation. That issue will be addressed in the context of discussing past research.

Drawbacks of the Psychoneuroimmunology Movement

Many have become excited at the prospect of drawing a theoretical and clinically relevant connection between psychological factors and cancer. However, preliminary evidence that there is some detectable relationship between psychosocial factors and the onset and progression of cancer has, unfortunately, had some unanticipated negative consequences. Unproven prevention and treatment methods capitalizing on the belief that attitude is a powerful immune mediator have already begun to proliferate and misrepresent current knowledge in the field. More importantly, cancer victims have reportedly been blamed and are blaming themselves for their diagnosis and ultimate demise. Some have come to believe that depression and anxiety about one's disease should be suppressed rather than expressed because of its potential ill effects. Others feel these emotions should in fact be expressed, because some studies have suggested that such expression is associated with better prognosis. While this is an understandable societal overreaction to what so far amount to preliminary scientific data, there is a need for increased sobriety on the part of investigators examining the stress–illness connection in cancer. This could in turn reduce these negative consequences.

There are many possible reasons why investigators and the general public need to believe in a strong link between stress and cancer. The tendency to exaggerate such a relationship may derive from the human motivation to perceive control and justice where little or none may exist. A belief that lowering stress can prevent or fight cancer fulfills a sense of personal control which can help those without cancer feel inoculated or at least prepared to fight the disease should it strike. The idea that the world is fair is also supported by a belief in a strong stress–cancer connection. Scarr (1985) has discussed the notion that 'knowledge' itself is constructed by the needs of the theorist, and that theory can in fact blind researchers to alternate interpretations of data. Certainly, studies which have examined the stress–illness connection in breast cancer have usually been compromised by methodological limitations that open the door to alternate interpretations of results. Examples of this are presented with the intention of encouraging future investigators in this area to consider and hopefully control for competing explanations of their data.

EARLY STUDIES IN BREAST CANCER

The Psychosomatic Movement

Initial excitement about the prospect of a clinically significant relationship between psychological factors and disease status in breast cancer was generated by a series of reports in the 1950s and 1960s. The central question has always been: 'Is there evidence that certain personality characteristics or certain attitudes or emotions are directly influential upon tumor growth?' This placed cancer among the 'psychosomatic illnesses' which were receiving extensive attention during that time. The empirical studies to substantiate the psychosomatic movement were, for the most part, significantly flawed by retrospective and cross-sectional methodologies that often had an unclear focus. In breast cancer, for example, Tarlau and Smalheiser (1951) used projective test data to compare women with cervical cancer to women with breast cancer. Extending far beyond the available data, the authors concluded that women with oral conflicts develop breast cancer while women with genital conflicts develop cervical cancer. In another study done around the same time, 40 women with breast cancer were assessed as being masochistic, sexually inhibited, unable to deal effectively with negative emotions, and showing signs of unresolved maternal conflict dating back to childhood (Bacon, Renneker and Cutler, 1952).

Life Event Studies

A common approach to studying the stress–illness connection has been the comparison of women who develop breast cancer to those who do not on scales designed to measure past life stress. The most consistently reported stressful event preceding the onset of cancer has been the loss of a loved one, either recently or during childhood (Greer and Morris, 1978). Nevertheless, even this relatively robust finding has met with equivocal support in the literature. For example, LeShan (1966) reported that loss of a major emotional relationship was contributory to cancer development. Yet in a controlled study reported in the very same journal volume, Muslin, Gyarfas and Pieper (1966) found no correlation between the loss of an important person, either during childhood or recently, and the onset of breast cancer.

These early studies of breast cancer are presented as examples of studies which relied upon cross-sectional and often retrospective data with patients who had active disease as a basis for conclusions about risk factors for development of cancer. Needless to say, research methodology has come a long way since these and other similar studies were published. However, it is important to recognize that many of the views of current researchers have been shaped by the beliefs espoused in these earlier investigations, and these views can hinder a scrutinizing and scientific inquiry into the problem.

THE IMPACT OF PSYCHONEUROIMMUNOLOGY

After a relatively quiet period during which psychosomatic theories of cancer development and progression fell out of favor, interest in psychosocial factors and cancer was again revived by progress in psychoneuroimmunology. Research outside of oncology had demonstrated that bereavement is associated with immune suppression (Bartrop *et al.*, 1977; Schleifer *et al.*, 1983), and the hypothesis seemed plausible that the anxiety and depression associated with cancer diagnosis and treatment could be immunocompromising as well.

Just prior to the above, there were animal data emerging to suggest that stress can enhance the incidence of tumor development in mice, particularly with spontaneous mammary gland carcinomas (Henry, Stephens and Watson, 1975; Riley, 1975). The work of Monjan and Collector (1977) had also provided animal data which supported a model of stress-induced alteration of immune function. Finally, in a study of major significance, Sklar and Anisman (1979) subjected mice to electric shock after implantation with syngenetic tumor cells. Tumor growth was significantly greater and norepinephrine levels were significantly lower in animals that were placed in the 'helpless' condition wherein they could not control their escape from shock. The combination of these two findings suggested that there is indeed a connection between the hormonal stress response (release of adrenal corticosterone) and immune suppression.

These connections drawn between stress, the hypothalamic–pituitary–adrenal axis and immunosuppression revived interest in studying the relationship between emotional response and the development of hormone-dependent tumors in humans. Subsequent human studies of this relationship in breast cancer are now reviewed.

Katz *et al.* (1970) studied emotional distress and cortisol production rates in 30 women awaiting breast biopsy. They found cortisol production rates to be significantly higher in women who reported greater distress and were rated as having inadequate defenses to deal with the stress of biopsy. Higher rates were also detected in the women who eventually received a diagnosis of malignancy. They did not, however, study the immune response of these 30 women, so conclusions about the association between heightened cortisol levels and immune suppression remain speculative.

In a ten-year follow-up study, Gorzynski *et al.* (1980) examined a subset of ten of the initial 30 women, using essentially the same methods. They found a surprising consistency in cortisol production rates within the ten women studied, suggesting that cortisol production may be a more stable marker over time than previously thought. They also determined, with this rather small sample (seven malignant; three benign), that the women who had malignant tumors continued to show higher cortisol levels, despite the fact that all subjects were disease-free at the time of assessment.

In another ten-year follow-up study of the same 30 women, Zumoff *et al.* (1982) reported that the factor of non-obesity at the time of mastectomy was a powerful predictor of ten-year disease-free survival. Non-obese women had significantly longer survival times. This is particularly important in the current context because emotional distress is known to be correlated with obesity, establishing this as a potential confounding variable that requires experimental control when looking at emotional distress as a predictor of tumor response. Not only is obesity associated with shorter survival after diagnosis of breast cancer, it is also a known risk factor for the disease itself.

EXPRESSION OF EMOTION: THE FIGHTING SPIRIT HYPOTHESIS

The longstanding notion that depression, social withdrawal, passivity and helplessness are psychological factors which predispose one to cancer and predict poor response to treatment have culminated in a popular notion that there is a 'cancer-prone' personality. Viewed from the opposite perspective, there has been increasing discussion of a 'fighting spirit' which, when present in a cancer patient, will enhance treatment response and increase survival time. The idea that a positive mental attitude and eagerness to fight one's disease is somehow immune-enhancing has received some support in women with breast cancer. This support has derived primarily from the work of the Faith Courtauld research group (Greer and Morris, 1975, 1978; Greer, Morris and Pettingale, 1979; Morris *et al.*, 1981; Pettingale *et al.*, 1985; Pettingale, Watson and Greer, 1984) and a study conducted at Johns Hopkins Hospital (Derogatis, Abeloff and Melisaratos, 1979).

The Courtauld studies

The basis for many of the conclusions of the Courtauld Unit research group of King's College in London was a study of 160 women admitted for breast tumor biopsy (Greer and Morris, 1975). Patients were interviewed and tested the day before surgery to obtain the following information: degree of depression, extraversion, neuroticism, intrapunitive hostility, extrapunitive hostility, occurrence of stressful life events, emotional response to life events, psychiatric history, frequency of expression of anger, interpersonal and marital adjustment, and work record. Of the 160 women, 69 were diagnosed with breast cancer, and it was the statistical comparisons of those 69 women to the 91 who had benign breast tumors that constituted the major study results.

The 69 women with breast cancer were found to express significantly less anger than the comparison group. Paradoxically, the women with cancer were also more likely to report a history of frequent temper outbursts. It is difficult to reconcile these apparently contradictory results, except to speculate that there is a pattern of emotionality in the women with breast cancer wherein they suppress anger as a predominant coping style, with resulting sporadic temper outbursts. The conclusion drawn from these data was that suppression of anger characterizes women who are vulnerable to breast cancer.

One of the major drawbacks of the above study, besides what is discussed in the next section, was that age was correlated with both diagnosis and suppression of anger: older women were more likely to have cancer and were more likely to suppress anger (Greer and Morris, 1975). Therefore, the correlation between diagnosis and personality may be spurious, with the true relationship being mediated by age. The authors, aware of this alternative possibility, split the sample into those above 50 and those below 50. In so doing, the correlation between suppression of anger and cancer diagnosis remained significant only in the women below 50 years of age. One must then ask if there is some reasonable psychoneuroimmunologic explanation for why there might be a stronger association between suppression of anger and cancer development in younger women. Without such a reasonable explanation, it seems more likely that there is some underlying confounding variable which would account for the differences.

Another noteworthy aspect of the study, again raised by some of the authors themselves in a later publication (Greer and Morris, 1978), was that despite the presence of a significant association between breast cancer and suppression of anger, there were no significant associations between breast cancer development and a host of other variables, including stressful life events, extraversion, depression, loss of a loved one, sexual inhibition, and denial as a characteristic response to stress. This then amounts to a study with a great deal of negative results which dispute earlier reports that suggest relationships between all of the above variables and cancer vulnerability.

Since the publication of these results, other studies have confirmed the tendency of women with breast cancer to show or express less emotion, particularly anxiety and anger, than healthy women (Jansen and Muenz, 1984; Morris *et al.*, 1981; Wirsching, 1982). This has led the Courtauld group to develop and validate a measure of emotional control, the Courtauld Emotional Control Scale (CECS), specifically for use in assessing this personality measure in cancer research (Pettingale, Watson and Greer, 1984; Watson and Greer, 1983). Future use of this measure will be critical in determining whether a construct of emotional control which predicts cancer initiation and progression can be operationalized.

The Courtauld group has reported two follow-up prospective studies of survival in women diagnosed with early stage breast cancer. The first was a five-year follow-up study which suggested that emotional response to diagnosis measured three months postoperatively was related to outcome (Greer, Morris and Pettingale, 1979). Those who reacted with 'denial' or a 'fighting spirit' were more likely to survive without recurrence than those who had reacted to diagnosis with 'stoic acceptance' or 'helplessness/hopelessness'. The four patient groups (denial, fighting spirit, stoic acceptance, hopeless/ helpless) were similar at diagnosis in terms of other prognostic indicators such as clinical stage, tumor size, histological grade, mammography, hormonal status and immunological status. With the exception of immunolog- ical status, equivalence across groups is a clear strength of the study. However, since the groups were similar also in immunological status, the results raise the question as to how one might explain later differential responses if not on the basis of differences in immune function.

The second follow-up study (Pettingale *et al.*, 1985) was conducted at ten years post diagnosis, on 57 women who had been tested as described earlier. Using a chi-square analysis, they again found that a favorable outcome was more common in the denial and fighting spirit groups than in the other two groups ($p=0.024$). A subsequent Cox regression with eight prognostic factors (age, menopausal status, clinical stage, type of operation, radiotherapy history, tumor size, histological grade and psychological response category) showed that psychological response category was the most powerful predictor of first recurrence ($p=0.008$), death from breast cancer ($p=0.003$) and death from any cause ($p=0.003$). The authors aptly caution that the results are based upon a small sample, with some of the cells containing fewer than two patients (Pettingale *et al.*, 1985). Also, histological examination of axillary nodes, a potentially valuable prognostic indicator, was unavailable in many of the patients. This and other unknown variables may covary with attitude towards illness and therefore represent a confound.

Related work

Cooper and colleagues (Cooper, Davies-Cooper and Faragher, 1986) studied 2163 women who underwent breast examinations at three different treatment centers in England. Women were evaluated after referral for breast examin- ation but before being told of their diagnosis. Patient variables of coping skill, social support, Type A behavior and recent life events were assessed with standardized instruments modified in ways to accommodate unique study and patient characteristics. Women were divided after diagnosis into four groups: cancer ($N=171$); cyst ($N=155$); benign breast disease ($N=1108$); and normal exam ($N=724$). The findings, reported as an extensive series of bivariate analyses, suggested that the women with breast cancer and those with cysts were significantly more likely to repress emotion, display poor coping skills and be more passive (as measured by the Type A scale) in the context of stress.

The greatest strength of the above study is its large sample size and its focus on only one site of potential disease (breast). However, it also has some weaknesses from which one can learn. First, it is a good example of a 'limited' prospective design in which assessment occurs before diagnosis, but there is no control for prediagnosis illness effects or subtly different communication patterns between patient and medical staff. This is discussed in more detail later.

A second issue, more specific to this study, is that there were significant differences between the four groups in age, with the cancer and cyst groups being older. Since some of these different personality patterns could arguably be determined by age differences, there is no certainty that the association between passivity and emotional suppression is a cancer-specific one. This is the same issue as that discussed with the Courtauld study (Greer and Morris, 1975). In a second analysis reported by Cooper *et al.* (1986), in which only women over 50 were studied, most of the differences between groups disappeared. As the authors themselves note, further reanalysis of their data is essential before a definitive link can be made between stress and breast cancer. A more appropriate analysis, which the authors are reportedly planning, would be a comprehensive multivariate approach which permits both control of Type I error rate inflation and statistical control for differences across groups in age. Incidentally, there were also differences across groups in marital status, occupational status, smoking and alcohol habits, and contraceptive use that would require control before a clear connection could be determined. Fortunately for the investigators, they appear to have a sufficient sample size to conduct this comprehensive analysis.

The Johns Hopkins study

An often cited study, this report examined 35 women with metastatic breast cancer at various points along the course of their disease (Derogatis, Abeloff and Melisaratos, 1979). Each woman was given a brief battery of self-report scales to measure mood and affect, was rated for overall adjustment by the study interviewer, and was rated for overall adjustment by the treating oncologist. The 35 women were then divided into those who died within one year ($N=13$) and those who survived longer than one year ($N=22$). The long-term survivors (more than one year) were reported to have higher psychological distress levels, especially depression and guilt, at the time of assessment than the short-term survivors. The authors conclude that the long-term survivors 'were distressed, and had measurable elevations in levels of anxiety and a sense of alienation; they were unhappy and they showed it in their moods' (Derogatis *et al.*, 1979, p. 1507).

On the surface, these results would appear to be consistent with those of the Courtauld group, inasmuch as expression of emotion was associated with longer survival time. However, as discussed elsewhere (Cella, 1985), there are a number of problems with this study which make most conclusions tentative. The 'elevated' scores which are used to suggest that high distress predicts good outcome were less than one standard deviation above the normal mean on eleven of twelve subscales on the psychological symptom inventory (Derogatis, 1977). Similarly, although the self-reported affect of the long-term survivors was indeed more 'negative' than the short-term survivors, the balance of affects reported by even the long-term survivors was in the *positive* range. It is therefore inaccurate to conclude that psychological distress or maladjustment is associated with long-term survival. Virtually all of the patients seemed to be functioning within a normal range on these scales.

Another issue regarding this study was that women were tested at different points in time relative to their diagnosis, confusing the biological disease and treatment response variables that may cause different psychological reactions. For example, 85 per cent of the short-term survivors had received prior chemotherapy, while this was true of only 55 per cent of the long-term survivors. Similarly, the short-term survivors were in chemotherapy for a much longer time prior to assessment ($M=407$ days) than the long-term survivors ($M=181$ days). These facts suggest that the short-term survivors had more advanced disease than the long-term survivors, a factor which itself could explain differences in survival. The authors do not report on any differences in number of positive axillary nodes across groups, but presumably the figure for the short-term survivors was higher, given that they received so much more chemotherapy. This again would be another underlying variable that could account for the group differences. Even if this were not the case, the mere impact of all the additional chemotherapy upon the short-term survivor group could be an underlying confounding variable which explained the differences in psychological response.

A failure to replicate

In an effort to improve upon problems of method and replicate the findings of Derogatis *et al.* (1979), Holland *et al.* (1986) in the Cancer and Leukemia Group B (CALGB) assessed 346 women with Stage II breast disease at the time of diagnosis. This study used a larger sample size, uniform pretreatment assessment at the time of diagnosis, and tight control over extent of chemotherapy received after assessment. All participants were entered into a clinical trial with treatment aims clearly defined according to protocol (CALGB Protocol μ8082). Participants completed the same symptom measure used in the Derogatis *et al.* (1979) study, and were followed for at least three years after diagnosis.

The above study failed to replicate the findings of Derogatis *et al.* (1979), which is particularly significant given the much larger sample. Psychological symptom scores did not predict disease-free survival or death when analyzed at the point of 106 (of 346) events ('event' was defined as either relapse or death). This was true when psychological symptom scores were analyzed separately or in conjunction with clinical prognostic variables such as number of positive axillary nodes or estrogen receptor status. There were some trends in the data that suggested there might be some weak relationship between psychological symptomatology at diagnosis and disease-free survival. Future analysis of this data set is needed to arrive at any firm conclusion about that, however.

LIMITATIONS OF PREVIOUS STUDIES

Overextrapolation From Animal Data

Many of the early studies in the psychoneuroimmunology of human breast cancer were stimulated by parallel developments with animals (Henry, Stephens and Watson, 1975; Monjan and Collector, 1977; Riley, 1975; Sklar and Anisman, 1979). These and other animal studies differed fundamentally from the human analogues in that they permitted far more experimental control over potentially confounding explanations for results. There has been a tendency on the part of investigators to derive hypotheses from animal models and test them in ways which do not really control for competing explanations. The result has been that theory *appears* to be supported when in fact it would be more truthful to say that the theory was not disconfirmed by the data.

Confounding Variables

Investigator zeal to confirm the presence of a psychosocial effect can blind one to the possibility of competing explanations of study results. For example, epidemiological studies, conducted around the same time as these initial human studies of the stress–illness connection, had defined several risk factors for occurrence of breast cancer. Some of these risk factors are: late age of first live birth, late marriage, late menopause, early menarche, obesity, history of cystic mastitis, family history of breast cancer, ionizing radiation, higher social class, and exogenous hormone use (MacMahon, Cole and Brown, 1973). Since many of these risk factors are associated with psychosocial factors that have been named as primary mediators of tumor initiation or response, the problem of potential confounding becomes clear. None of these early studies has controlled for these potentially confounding factors, so their results and conclusions must be considered tentative.

Deemphasis of Negative or Non-Confirmatory Results

It is commonly noted that studies reporting negative results are less likely to be submitted for publication and, when submitted, less likely to be accepted. It seems equally true that investigators have a tendency to remember the positive results of a study which does get reported. For example, most researchers and clinicians in this area of study will tell you that the Courtauld research group has shown that reduced expression of emotion is associated with cancer vulnerability. However, few will add that the same research data failed to replicate over half a dozen other factors previously identified as associated with cancer vulnerability. These other factors tend to remain associated with the investigators who succeeded in detecting an association. The result can be an honest exaggeration of the true relationship between psychological factors and cancer, or at least of the generalizability of findings.

Population Base Rate of Cancer

A commonly discussed drawback of any prospective epidemiological study of breast cancer incidence is the low base rate of incidence in the general population. Thousands of women must be studied over decades in order to get a truly prospective view of the question of cancer incidence. Rarely is such a study feasible. Shekelle *et al.* (1981) prospectively studied 2020 employees of the Western Electric Company and documented that high MMPI depression scores were indeed associated with risk of cancer in a seventeen-year follow up. Other large-scale epidemiological studies of cancer incidence include Hagnell's (1966) Swedish study and the study of Thomas and McCabe (1980) in the United States. These two studies have entered thousands of participants and yet have accumulated just over 100 total cancer cases for analysis. For example, after ten years, Hagnell's (1966) study of 2550 people provided only nine cases of breast cancer for analysis. Because of this limitation, large epidemiological studies have looked at *overall* cancer incidence rather than vulnerability to site-specific malignancies such as breast cancer. This may serve to dilute an effect, because psychosocial vulnerability is probably site-specific.

Limited Prospective Studies

Frequently, investigators have opted to use a limited prospective design to circumvent the problem in managing and supporting fully prospective studies, and to enable the study of one disease site. This design typically assesses people at some time during a medical work-up for cancer, before the diagnosis is known (e.g. Cooper, Davies-Cooper and Faragher, 1986; Greer and

Morris, 1975; Katz *et al.*, 1970). While this allows for prediagnosis assessment for prediction of cancer versus non-cancer cases, there are some major drawbacks. First, since diagnosis does not mark the time at which the disease begins exerting its impact upon the body, one can never be certain that the individuals with cancer have not already begun to experience some disease-related emotional response. Etiology of such a response could be physical (e.g. paraneoplastic syndrome) or psychological (e.g. sensing the reaction of medical staff to a probable cancer diagnosis). A second problem with limited prospective designs is that correlation cannot be construed as causality, since it is unclear which event (cancer or distress) predates the other.

RECENT TRENDS IN BREAST CANCER RESEARCH

In some respects, the limitations of the early studies of the stress–illness connection in human breast cancer have been addressed and partially corrected in more recent studies. Having learned from the inevitable mistakes and oversights of earlier studies, some of the newer research in this area has provided a more comprehensive view of the picture. Nevertheless, there continue to be limitations in method evident in these more recent studies, largely due to the complexity of the problem being studied and the impossibility of conducting true experimental research in humans. A review of three selected recent studies of the stress–illness connection in breast cancer follows.

The National Institutes of Health (NIH) study

As emphasized by Levy *et al.* (1985), the next important step in the study of psychological factors and cancer involves the specification of 'biological mediating mechanisms linking behavior with biological risk status' (p. 111). Towards that end, a recent NIH study has begun to examine the relationship between positive axillary node status (the best known predictor of outcome in breast cancer) and natural killer (NK) cell activity in women with breast cancer (Levy *et al.*, 1985). Indeed, in that study of 75 women with Stage I or II breast cancer, NK activity was reduced in women with more positive nodes ($p<0.01$). In the current context, this is useful information because it permits some justification for assuming that immunity is indeed measurably compromised in the time period following diagnosis, and that this compromised immunity is potentially meaningful in terms of tumor response. Although the long-term data for this NIH study are not yet known, cross-sectional studies of psychological differences associated with reduced NK activity have been made available (Levy *et al.*, 1985).

The psychological symptom checklist and observer rating scale were the same ones used by Derogatis, Abeloff and Melisaratos (1979) and Holland *et al.* (1986). This study also used the Profile of Mood States (POMS; McNair, Lorr and Droppleman, 1971) to measure current mood. In this preliminary cross-sectional report, the authors compared psychological data to immune data (NK activity) and clinical prognostic data (nodal status). The SCL-90-R summary score, identified as significant in the Derogatis *et al.* (1979) study, did not contribute significant explanatory power to either of the two outcome measures. In the prediction of NK activity, three factors emerged as significant, accounting for 51 per cent of the variance: global rating of adjustment (those rated as better adjusted had *lower* NK activity); social support (reduced support was associated with lower NK activity); and fatigue (higher scores were associated with lower NK activity).

It is unfortunate that the authors chose to select the Fatigue scale over Depression as the POMS variable to enter into the regression analysis. Fatigue items on the POMS are very physically laden, and could be indicative of reduced performance status or general ill health, where the same interpretation is less tenable with the POMS Depression scale. The result is that the report leaves open the interpretation that the relationship between POMS Fatigue and NK activity is not a psycho-physical one but a physico-physical one. The fact that the POMS Fatigue and Depression subscales are highly intercorrelated (0.76 in their sample) suggests that selection of the Depression scale might have yielded similar results. The problem then is that interpretation of this relationship becomes very subjective inasmuch as one could refer to an association between apathy and reduced NK activity, or between expressed emotion (i.e. expression of depression) and reduced NK activity. The same results could lead to two equally valid but apparently contradictory conclusions. If one went with the interpretation that expression of depression was associated with immune suppression, this would run counter to the data of the Courtauld group and the Derogatis *et al.* (1979) study. Further analysis of Levy *et al.*'s (1985) data could examine this issue. At present, however, with knowledge of what has been reported, it is unclear whether a reliable connection between psychological state and immune function, as it relates to breast cancer prognosis, has been established.

The Roswell Park study

A very different approach to the question of stress and breast cancer progression was conducted by Marshall and Funch (1983). In 1979, they reviewed 283 known deaths out of a pool of 353 women who had been diagnosed with primary breast cancer between 1958 and 1960. Each patient had been asked about the occurrence of a number of traumatic events in the five years preceding first recognition of symptoms. Marital status, religious involvement and a variety of other crude indicators of the depth of social support structure were also ascertained. In general, results supported the hypothesis that preillness social stress is associated with shorter survival time. However, the single most powerful predictor of survival was stage at diagnosis, accounting for 15–20 per cent of the variance of survival time. After that, an additional 9 per cent of the variance was explained by social indicators, but *only* in the group of women younger than 46 years of age. Social indicators did not add explanatory power in the older women.

The authors point out that their social indicators are crude and, as such, may underestimate the effects of social support upon survival. On the other hand, there were no available data on the psychological state of the women at the time of assessment, so there was no way the investigators could control for unknown concurrent variables such as distress or even subjective stress level. Even some 'standard', equally crude sociological variables, such as social class and income, appeared unavailable to the investigators. Nevertheless, the fact that global sociological parameters can predict length of survival, even if not fully controlled and only in younger women, gives reason to encourage further elaboration of this area in future studies.

The University of Pennsylvania study

Cassileth *et al.* (1985) reported a prospective follow-up study of 204 patients with unresectable cancers (pancreatic, gastric, lung, colorectal and glioma) and 155 patients with Stage I or II melanoma or Stage II breast cancer. The former group ('Group 1') was assessed for survival time, while the latter ('Group 2') was assessed for time to recurrence. Predictor variables were a composite of seven psychosocial characteristics reported in previous investigations as predictive of longevity or survival in cancer: social ties, marital history, job satisfaction, use of psychotropic drugs, general life satisfaction, subjective health evaluation, and hopelessness/helplessness. The strengths of the study are its comprehensive approach to psychosocial variables and its relatively large sample size. The major weaknesses of the study are its selection of primarily uncurable diseases (Group 1), where the effect of psychosocial variables is likely to be least evident (Levy, 1985), and the selection of measures.

Analysis of all 359 patients revealed that psychosocial factors, taken individually and in combination, were uncorrelated with other clinical variables and had no influence upon length of survival or time to relapse. The authors conclude: 'the biology of the disease appears to predominate and to override the potential influence of life-style and psychosocial variables once the disease process is established' (Cassileth *et al.*, 1985, p. 1551). Although this is unsurprising in the unresectable tumor group, the results with patients in the melanoma and breast cancer group run counter to many previous reports.

The results of the above study indeed reflect the absence of a strong, clearly detectable psychosocial effect upon the progression of breast cancer (among other sites). However, there is a problem with measurement reliability and sophistication which must be addressed. Until such time, it is advisable that the investigator's mind remain open about the possibility of a psychosocial effect upon tumor progression. Cassileth *et al.* (1985) chose to measure most of the seven psychosocial attributes with very brief, often unvalidated single-item measures. One well-validated measure of depression was included, however. The decision to use relatively unvalidated assessment potentially compromises the certainty that the constructs under question were adequately or accurately assessed. If the constructs were in fact unreliably measured, then the statistical power of the tests was compromised. Also, the respondents were at times asked to retrospectively rate their premorbid state, which could introduce an unknown source of response bias.

This study failed to confirm the hypothesis of psychosocial correlates of disease progression. It did so with a creative approach to data collection that carried some risks of Type II error (failure to detect a significant effect). Nevertheless, it is likely that if the impact of psychosocial variables named in previous studies is strong, even a crude effort at measuring these variables would turn up some significant findings. This supports the commonly held view mentioned at the beginning of this chapter: that if there is an impact of psychosocial variables, it is likely to be very small relative to the impact of other clinical and known prognostic variables.

CONCLUSION

The application of psychoneuroimmunology to the study of breast cancer is controversial, exciting and, most of all, at a very early stage of development. The fact that three separate studies with differing methodologies (Cooper, Davies Cooper and Faragher, 1986; Greer and Morris, 1975; Marshall and Funch, 1983) all showed evidence to suggest that a psychoneuroimmunological effect is more likely to be present in younger (premenopausal) women is an observation that suggests the need for further study. New and more comprehensive approaches to examining this and other interesting questions are necessary to help advance the current state of knowledge in the area. Studies must control for confounding variables such as weight, age and nodal status. Investigators are encouraged to approach the area enthusiastically but with a skeptical eye that is aware of potential errors of interpretation and overextrapolation of results. Improved measurement strategies and better coordination of psychological and biological response assessment promise to add valuable data in future studies.

REFERENCES

Ader, R. (Ed.) (1981). *Psychoneuroimmunology*, Academic Press, Orlando, Fl.

Bacon, C. L., Renneker, R., and Cutler, M. A. (1952). A psychosomatic survey of cancer of the breast, *Psychosom. Med.*, **14**, 453–460.

Bartrop, R. W., Lazarus, L., Luckhurst, E., Kiloh, L. G., and Penny, R. (1977). Depressed lymphocyte function after bereavement, *Lancet*, **1**, 834–836.

Cassileth, B. R., Lusk, E. J., Miller, D. S., Brown, L. L., and Miller, C. (1985). Psychosocial correlates of survival in advanced malignant disease? *N. Eng. J. Med.*, **312**, 1551–1555.

Cella, D. F. (1985). Psychological adjustment and cancer outcome: Levy versus Taylor, *Am. Psychol.*, **40**, 1275–1276.

Cooper, C. L., Davies-Cooper, R. F., and Faragher, E. B. (1986). A prospective study of the relationship between breast cancer and life events, Type A behaviour, social support and coping skills, *Stress Med.*, **2**, 271–277.

Cox, T., and MacKay, C. (1982). Psychosocial factors and psychophysiological mechanisms in the aetiology and development of cancers, *Soc. Sci. Med.*, **16**, 381–396.

Derogatis, L. R. (1977). *Administration, Scoring and Procedures Manual for the SCL-90-R*, Clinical Psychometrics Research, Baltimore.

Derogatis, L. R., Abeloff, M. D., and Melisaratos, N. (1979). Psychological coping mechanisms and survival time in breast cancer, *J. Am. Med. Assoc.*, **242**, 1504–1508.

Fox, B. H. (1983). Current theory of psychogenic effects on cancer incidence and prognosis, *J. Psychosoc. Oncol.*, **1**, 1, 17–31.

Gorzynski, J. G., Holland, J., Katz, J. L., Weiner, H., Zumoff, B., Fukishima, D., and Levin, J. (1980). Stability of ego defenses and endocrine responses in women prior to breast biopsy and ten years later, *Psychosom. Med.*, **42**, 323–328.

Greer, S., and Morris, T. (1975). Psychological attributes of women who develop breast cancer: A controlled study, *J. Psychosom. Res.*, **19**, 147–153.

Greer, S., and Morris, T. (1978). The study of psychological factors in breast cancer: problems of method, *Soc. Sci. Med.*, **12** (3A), 129–134.

Greer, S., Morris, T., and Pettingale, K. W. (1979). Psychological response to breast cancer: effect on outcome, *Lancet*, **ii**, 785–787.

Hagnell, O. (1966). The premorbid personality of persons who develop cancer in a total population investigated in 1947 and 1957, *Ann. NY Acad. Sci.*, **125**, 846–855.

Henry, J. P., Stephens, P. M., and Watson, F. M. C. (1975). Force breeding, social disorder and mammary tumor formation in CBA/USC mouse colonies: A pilot study, *Psychosom. Med.*, **37**, 277–283.

Holland, J. C., Korzun, A. H., Tross, S., Cella, D. F., Norton, L., and Wood, W., for Cancer and Leukemia Group B. (1986). Psychosocial factors and disease-free survival (DFS) in stage II breast carcinoma, *Proc. ASCO*, **5**, 237 (μ928).

Jansen, M. A., and Muenz, L. R. (1984). A retrospective study of personality variables associated with fibrocystic disease and breast cancer, *J. Psychosom. Res.*, **28**, 35–42.

Jemmott, J. B., and Locke, S. E. (1984). Psychosocial factors, immunologic mediation, and human susceptibility to infectious diseases: How much do we know? *Psychol Bull.*, **95**(1), 78–108.

Katz, J. L., Ackman, P., Rothwax, Y., Sacher, E. J., Weiner, H., Hellman, L., and Gallagher, T. F. (1970). Psychoendocrine aspects of cancer of the breast, *Psychosom. Med.*, **32**, 1–18.

LeShan, L. (1966). An emotional life-history pattern associated with neoplastic disease, *Ann. NY Acad. Sci.*, **125**, 780–793.

Levy, S. M. (1985). *Behavior and Cancer*, Jossey-Bass, San Francisco.

Levy, S. M., Herberman, R. B., Maluish, A. M., Schlien, B., and Lippman, M. (1985). Prognostic risk assessment in primary breast cancer by behavioral and immunological parameters, *Health Psychol.*, **4**, 2, 99–113.

MacMahon, B., Cole, P., and Brown, J. (1973). Etiology of human breast cancer: A review, *J. Nat. Cancer. Inst.*, **50**, 21–42.

Marshall, J. R., and Funch, D. P. (1983). Social environment and breast cancer: A cohort analysis of patient survival, *Cancer*, **52**, 1546–1550.

McNair, D., Lorr, M., and Droppleman, L. (1971). *EITS manual for the Profile of Mood States*, Educational and Industrial Testing Service, San Diego.

Monjan, A., and Collector, M. (1977). Stress-induced modulation of immune function, *Science*, **196**, 307–308.

Morris, T., Greer, S., Pettingale, K. W., and Watson, M. (1981). Patterns of expression of anger and their psychological correlates in women with breast cancer, *J. Psychosom. Res.*, **25**, 111–117.

Muslin, H. L., Gyarfas, K., and Pieper, W. J. (1966). Separation experience and cancer of the breast, *Ann. NY Acad. Sci.*, **125**, 802–806.

Pettingale, K. W., Morris, T., Greer, S., and Haybittle, J. L. (1985). Mental attitudes to cancer: an additional prognostic factor, *Lancet*, **i**, 750.

Pettingale, K. W., Watson, M., and Greer, S. (1984). The validity of emotional control as a trait in breast cancer patients, *J. Psychosoc. Oncol.*, **2** (3/4), 21–30.

Riley, V. (1975). Mouse mammary tumors: Alteration of incidence as apparent function of stress, *Science*, **189**, 465–467.

Scarr, S. (1985). Constructing psychology: making facts and fables for our times, *Am. Psychol.*, **40**, 499–512.

Schleifer, S. J., Keller, S. E., Camerino, M., Thornton, J. C., and Stein, M. (1983). Suppression of lymphocyte stimulation following bereavement, *J. Am. Med. Assoc.*, **250**, 374–377.

Shekelle, R. B., Raynor, W. J., Ostfeld, A. M., Garron, D. C., Bieliauskas, L. A., Liu, S. C., Maliza, C., and Paul, O. (1981). Psychological depression and 17-year risk of death from cancer, *Psychosom. Med.*, **43**, 117–125.

Sklar, L. S., and Anisman, H. (1979). Stress and coping factors influence tumor growth, *Science*, **205**, 513–515.

Sklar, L. S., and Anisman, H. (1981). Stress and cancer, *Psychol. Bull.*, **89** (3), 369–406.

Tarlau, M., and Smalheiser, I. (1951). Personality patterns in patients with malignant tumors of the breast and cervix, *Psychosom. Med.*, **13**, 117–121.

Thomas, C. B., and McCabe, O. L. (1980). Precursors of premature disease and death: Habits of nervous tension, *Johns Hopkins Med. J.*, **147**, 137–145.

Watson, M., and Greer, S. (1983). Development of a questionnaire measure of emotional control, *J. Psychosom. Res.*, **27**, 299–305.

Wirsching, M. (1982). Psychological identification of breast cancer patients before biopsy, *J. Psychosom. Res.*, **26**, 1–10.

Zumoff, B., Gorzynski, J. G., Katz, J. L., Weiner, H., Levin, J., Holland, J., and Fukishima, D. K. (1982). Nonobesity at the time of mastectomy is highly predictive of 10-year disease-free survival in women with breast cancer, *Anticancer Res.*, **2**, 59–62.

Index